MEDPRO WRITERS

PHARMACOLOGY AND PHYSIOLOGY FOR LUMBAR EPIDURAL ANESTHESIA (FOUNDATION AND CLINICAL APPLICATION)

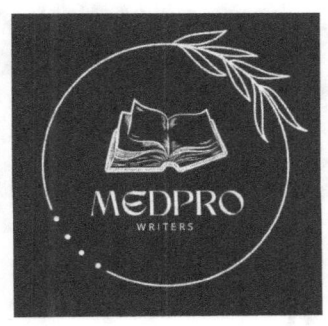

Copyright © 2024 by MedPro Writers

All rights reserved. No part of this publication may be reproduced, stored or transmitted in any form or by any means, electronic, mechanical, photocopying, recording, scanning, or otherwise without written permission from the publisher. It is illegal to copy this book, post it to a website, or distribute it by any other means without permission.

MedPro Writers asserts the moral right to be identified as the author of this work.

First edition

ISBN: 9798327944886

This book was professionally typeset on Reedsy. Find out more at reedsy.com

Contents

Chapter 1	1
Chapter 2	11
Chapter 3	29
Chapter 4	43
Chapter 5	73
Chapter 6	88
Chapter 7	110
Chapter 8	138
Chapter 9	151
Chapter 10	167
Chapter 11	177
Chapter 12	187
Chapter 13	202
Chapter 14	214
Chapter 15	226
Chapter 16	237

Chapter 1

INTRODUCTION TO LUMBAR EPIDURAL ANESTHESIA

1.1. Definition and Overview

Lumbar epidural anesthesia stands as a quiet guardian, on the brink of relief from pain, in the darkened sanctuary of the operating room, where the muted murmurs of expectation blend with the aroma of antiseptic. In this precise balance between pharmacology and physiology, the anesthesiologist orchestrates a symphony of sensations to expose the essence of lumbar epidural anesthesia.Lumbar epidural anesthesia is essentially a master class in modulation, a well orchestrated waltz of molecules and membranes. Characterized by its careful injection into the lumbar epidural region, a holy area between the bony vertebrae and the dural sac, this method signals a new era in pain treatment. An oasis of peace is created inside the lumbar epidural region, a haven for individuals entangled by the tangles of agony in the otherwise parched desert of suffering.Exploring the maze of neuroanatomy and pharmacokinetics is the path to understanding lumbar epidural anesthesia. Arcane rites of drug distribution give birth to the alchemy of analgesia, setting out on a journey full of intricacy and depth. As the symphony of feeling gives way to the subdued whispers of anesthesia, the lines between awareness and oblivion blur inside this sacred zone.

However, lumbar epidural anesthesia is a demonstration of the unyielding determination of the human spirit—it is more than just a method of pain relief. Lumbar epidural anesthesia, from its modest beginnings in medical history to its present-day pinnacle, is a testament to the never-ending pursuit of therapeutic intervention perfection. It is a monument to the daring of visionaries who dared to question the established dogmas of pain treatment, establishing new roads among the wilderness of suffering.

In the broad tapestry of medical knowledge, lumbar epidural anesthesia appears as a light of hope among the shadows of misery. It is a tribute to the transformational power of knowledge, lighting the route towards a future when suffering is not just endured, but vanquished—a future where the promise of peace beckons, just beyond the threshold of awareness.

1.2. Historical Background

To trace the roots of lumbar epidural anesthesia is to go on a trip through the annals of medical history, where the seeds of invention were sowed amongst the rich soil of human curiosity. Like a history spreading over time's length, the birth of this approach finds resonance in the pioneering initiatives of brave minds who dared to confront the established dogmas of pain treatment.The narrative starts in the closing years of the 19th century, against the background of a rapidly expanding medical scene. It was here, among the growing city of Berlin, that the scene was prepared for a major confrontation between science and pain. August Bier, a light of his day, was poised upon the verge of discovery, his eyes set upon the mysterious world of spinal anesthesia.In the year 1898, Bier started upon a series of ambitious investigations, traveling where few had ventured to tread—the world of the spinal canal. With painstaking accuracy, he delivered a cocaine solution into the subarachnoid space of a consenting volunteer, ushering in a new era in the annals of anesthesia. The outcome was nothing short of miraculous—the volunteer remained cognizant and attentive, but free of pain—a monument to the transformational power of lumbar spinal anesthesia.

Yet, it was not until the start of the 20th century that lumbar epidural anesthesia finally came into its own, spurred by the pioneering work of Achille Dogliotti. Building upon Bier's fundamental work, Dogliotti developed the procedure, refining the art of lumbar epidural anesthesia with exceptional accuracy. His revolutionary research provided the framework for modern-day practice, pointing the route towards a future when pain would be vanquished, not only endured.

From these basic beginnings sprang a revolution in the realm of pain treatment, as lumbar epidural anesthesia became a cornerstone of contemporary medical practice. With each passing decade, the approach expanded and thrived, spurred by the unrelenting march of scientific advancement. Today, lumbar epidural anesthesia stands as a tribute to the resilient spirit of human inquiry, a light of hope among the shadows of misery.

1.3. Indications and Contraindications

In the sophisticated arithmetic of medical decision-making, the delineation of criteria and contraindications for lumbar epidural anesthesia acquires a crucial relevance, leading the physician through the labyrinthine corridors of therapeutic choice. Like a compass amid the maelstrom of uncertainty, these guiding principles light the road towards optimum patient care, diverting the course away from treacherous shoals towards the beaches of safety and effectiveness.Indications for lumbar epidural anesthesia encompass a wide range of clinical circumstances, ranging from the treatment of acute surgical pain to the reduction of persistent neuropathic discomfort. Whether it is the palliation of labor pains or the amelioration of postoperative agony, lumbar epidural anesthesia stands as a steadfast ally in the armory of pain management, providing consolation to the suffering and rest to the weary.

Yet, among the tapestry of therapeutic promise, lay the shadows of contraindications, casting their foreboding shape over the canvas of clinical decision-making. From the specter of coagulopathy to the fear of local infection, these contraindications function as sentinels, protecting the gates against the entry of harm. It is through the discerning eye of the physician that the delicate balance between risk and reward is established, ensuring that the beacon of lumbar epidural anesthesia remains a guiding light amongst the stormy seas of medical practice.In the area of obstetrics, lumbar epidural anesthesia has evolved as a cornerstone of contemporary delivery, affording pregnant women a break from the agony of labor. The approach, when appropriately performed, offers significant pain treatment without compromising mother or fetal well-being. However, care must be used in some conditions, including as cases of maternal coagulopathy or severe hypotension, when the hazards may exceed the benefits.

Similarly, in the field of orthopedic surgery, lumbar epidural anesthesia has changed the treatment of postoperative pain, providing patients a smoother transition from the operating table to recovery. Yet, in patients with spinal abnormalities or pre-existing neurological disorders, great attention must be given to the possible dangers of epidural implantation, since unintentional harm to neural structures may lead to disastrous outcomes.Beyond the areas of obstetrics and orthopedics, lumbar epidural anesthesia finds applicability in a plethora of therapeutic circumstances, from the treatment of persistent back pain to the palliation of terminal disease. Yet, with each indication comes a comparable set of contraindications, needing a thoughtful evaluation of risk and reward.

In the hands of a qualified practitioner, lumbar epidural anesthesia is a formidable instrument in the armamentarium of contemporary medicine, affording patients a reprieve from the ravages of pain. Yet, like any therapeutic intervention, it is not without its hazards. It is through the painstaking application of knowledge and expertise that the clinician navigates the hazardous seas of doubt, bringing the patient towards the beaches of healing with wisdom and compassion.

1.4. Anatomy and Physiology of the Lumbar Epidural Space

To appreciate the nuances of lumbar epidural anesthesia, one must first travel the labyrinthine tunnels of spinal anatomy, where the lumbar epidural space appears as a critical nexus in the world of pain regulation. Nestled amidst the spinal column and the dural sac, this anatomical sanctuary conceals the potential for substantial therapeutic intervention, affording a portal to the world of analgesia.The lumbar epidural space, a fusiform reservoir of adipose tissue and loose connective fibers, has a key location inside the spinal canal, stretching from the lower thoracic to the sacral region. Bounded dorsally by the ligamentum flavum and ventrally by the posterior longitudinal ligament, the lumbar epidural space constitutes a sanctuary of sorts, shielding the fragile neural structures from the vagaries of mechanical injury.

Yet, it is not only the physical dimensions of the lumbar epidural region that give it receptive to therapeutic intervention—it is the dynamic interplay of physiological factors that endow it with its analgesic potential. Within this holy region, a delicate balance is achieved between the influx and outflow of cerebrospinal fluid, as the ebb and flow of physiologic currents create the geometry of the lumbar epidural space.From a pharmacological standpoint, the lumbar epidural region is a genuine pharmacokinetic playground, where the complex rituals of drug transport find fertile ground for investigation. With each infusion of anesthetic drug, a delicate dance occurs, as molecules navigate the labyrinthine pathways of adipose tissue and capillary beds, finding their elusive targets among the sea of brain tissue.It is within this dynamic environment that the magic of lumbar epidural anesthesia unfolds, as the careful administration of local anesthetics and adjuvants delivers a symphony of analgesia, choreographed with precision. From the somatic fibers of the dorsal root ganglia to the autonomic plexuses of the sympathetic chain, the neurological pathways of pain are trapped inside the soft embrace of anesthesia, as the borders between awareness and forgetfulness blur.

Yet, within the grandeur of pharmacological modulation, lay the shadows of possible risk, as the casual administration of epidural anesthetic may give birth to unexpected effects. From the danger of unintended dural puncture to the potential of systemic toxicity, the risks of lumbar epidural anesthesia loom large, casting a cloud over the landscape of therapeutic promise.

It is via the discerning eye of the anesthesiologist that the delicate balance between risk and reward is established, as the art of lumbar epidural anesthesia emerges amongst the tapestry of spinal anatomy and physiology. With each needle puncture and infusion of medicine, a symphony of feeling is arranged, providing consolation to the ailing and rest to the weary.

1.5. Techniques of Lumbar Epidural Anesthesia

Within the field of lumbar epidural anesthesia, a multiplicity of procedures and approaches exist, each suited to the particular demands and anatomical concerns of the individual patient. From the conventional landmark-based strategy to the cutting-edge ultrasound-guided technique, the landscape of lumbar epidural anesthesia is as broad as it is dynamic.The traditional landmark-based approach, also known as the loss of resistance technique, is a time-honored method of lumbar epidural anesthesia, whereby the anesthesiologist relies upon tactile input to locate the epidural space. Using a specialist epidural needle outfitted with a loss of resistance syringe, the physician navigates the bony landmarks of the lumbar spine, seeking the elusive pop that signals admission into the epidural space.While the landmark-based strategy has lasted the test of time, it is not without its limits. Variability in patient anatomy and operator expertise may lead to inadequate needle placement, increasing the risk of unintentional dural puncture or failure block. As such, other procedures have arisen in recent years, giving increased precision and effectiveness in the administration of lumbar epidural anesthetic.

One such method is the paramedian approach, whereby the needle is injected lateral to the midline, targeting the epidural space at a position away from the midline tissues. This method provides various benefits over the standard midline approach, including lower risk of dural puncture and enhanced visibility of the epidural area on imaging investigations.In recent years, the development of ultrasound technology has transformed the practice of lumbar epidural anesthesia, enabling real-time view of anatomical structures and needle trajectory. With the use of ultrasound guidance, the anesthesiologist may accurately define the epidural space and monitor the distribution of local anesthesia with unparalleled precision. This strategy has been demonstrated to enhance block success rates and decrease problems compared to standard landmark-based procedures.

Beyond the area of needle insertion, the choice of drug and adjuncts plays a vital role in the effectiveness of lumbar epidural anesthesia. Local anesthetics such as bupivacaine and ropivacaine are often utilized for their powerful analgesic qualities, while adjuncts such as opioids and adjuvants may be given to increase block length and quality.

In summary, lumbar epidural anesthesia comprises a varied variety of methods and procedures, each with its own specific benefits and limits. From the traditional landmark-based method to the cutting-edge ultrasound-guided technique, the landscape of lumbar epidural anesthesia continues to advance, driven by the constant quest of perfection in the world of pain management.

1.6. Complications and Adverse Effects

Despite its efficiency in delivering pain relief, lumbar epidural anesthesia is not without its hazards, since problems and side effects may arise, ranging from small nuisances to life-threatening situations. Understanding these possible problems is critical for the safe and successful administration of lumbar epidural anesthesia, enabling practitioners to limit risk and enhance patient outcomes. One of the most frequent risks associated with lumbar epidural anesthesia is unintended dural puncture, which may occur during needle insertion. This may lead to release of CSF fluid and subsequent development of post-dural puncture headache—a debilitating disorder characterized by intense headache aggravated by upright position. While most instances heal spontaneously with conservative care, severe or refractory cases may need epidural blood patching to plug the dural hole and reduce symptoms.

In addition to dural puncture, additional problems connected with lumbar epidural anesthesia include epidural hematoma, epidural abscess, and unintentional intravascular injection. Epidural hematoma—an uncommon but potentially severe complication—may arise related to damage to the epidural vasculature, leading to compression of neural structures and consequent neurological impairments. Similarly, epidural abscess—a localized accumulation of pus inside the epidural space—may occur as a consequence of bacterial infection during needle placement or catheter insertion. Prompt detection and treatment of these consequences are crucial to avoid irreparable neuronal impairment and systemic infection. Inadvertent intravascular injection is another possible consequence of lumbar epidural anesthesia, especially when delivering significant amounts of local anesthetic or opioid. Injection into a blood artery may lead to systemic toxicity, presenting as central nervous system depression, cardiovascular collapse, and respiratory arrest. Vigilant monitoring and timely action are important to limit the danger of systemic toxicity and maintain patient safety.

In addition to these immediate difficulties, lumbar epidural anesthesia may also be linked with a number of side effects, including pruritus, urine retention, and temporary neurologic signs. Pruritus—a typical adverse effect of neuraxial opioids—may develop related to opioid-induced histamine release, resulting in acute itching of the skin. While normally self-limiting, severe or chronic episodes may need pharmaceutical intervention with antihistamines or opioid antagonists.

Similarly, urine retention—a result of sympathetic blockade—may develop during lumbar epidural anesthesia, especially in patients having lower extremities surgery or receiving high-dose opioids. Timely intervention with bladder catheterization or pharmacological medications may be essential to treat urine retention and avoid bladder distention.

Transient neurologic symptoms—a poorly understood phenomena characterized by radicular pain, dysesthesia, and motor weakness—may develop during lumbar epidural anesthesia, especially with the administration of hyperbaric local anesthetics. While normally self-limiting and benign, transitory neurologic symptoms may cause substantial pain and concern for individuals. Education and reassurance are vital to reduce patient fears and avoid unneeded measures.

In summary, lumbar epidural anesthesia is a powerful instrument in the armamentarium of pain management, delivering excellent relief for a broad variety of surgical and obstetric operations. However, like any medical intervention, it is not without its hazards, and physicians must stay attentive for any problems and unpleasant consequences. With careful patient selection, thorough technique, and timely diagnosis of adverse events, lumbar epidural anesthesia may be provided safely and efficiently, reducing pain and enhancing patient results.

1.7. Future Directions and Emerging Technologies

As the discipline of lumbar epidural anesthesia continues to expand, so too do the technology and procedures utilized in its administration. From revolutionary medication formulations to cutting-edge imaging technologies, the future offers immense potential for the progress of pain treatment and patient care. One area of ongoing study is the development of long-acting local anesthetics and innovative drug delivery methods, aiming at lengthening the duration of pain treatment and lowering the need for additional analgesics. Liposomal preparations of bupivacaine, for example, have been demonstrated to increase the duration of sensory blocking after epidural injection, giving prospective advantages for patients undergoing major surgery or enduring chronic pain. In addition to drug discovery, breakthroughs in imaging technology are altering the practice of lumbar epidural anesthesia, allowing for real-time viewing of needle insertion and medication dissemination. Fluoroscopy-guided epidural injections, for example, provide improved accuracy and precision compared to conventional landmark-based procedures, minimizing the risk of problems and enhancing block quality.

Similarly, ultrasound-guided lumbar puncture and epidural catheter insertion have emerged as useful tools in the armamentarium of the anesthesiologist, allowing real-time view of anatomical structures and needle trajectory. With the use of ultrasound guidance, doctors may properly identify the epidural area and monitor the dissemination of medicine, guaranteeing optimum block placement and effectiveness. Beyond the area of procedural technique, new technologies like virtual reality and augmented reality show considerable potential for boosting patient comfort and satisfaction during lumbar epidural anesthesia. By immersing patients in immersive virtual worlds or layering digital information onto their surroundings, doctors may divert patients from procedural pain and minimize anxiety, permitting easier epidural insertion and block administration.

In summary, the future of lumbar epidural anesthesia is bright, with breakthroughs in medication research, imaging technology, and patient interaction ready to alter the profession of pain management. By embracing these advancements and keeping watchful for evolving trends and technology, physicians may continue to give safe, effective, and compassionate care to patients in need.

Chapter 2

ANATOMY RELEVANT TO LUMBAR EPIDURAL ANESTHESIA

2.1. Spinal Column Anatomy

In the broad expanse of human anatomy, the spinal column appears as a magnificent pillar, a tribute to the meticulous workmanship of evolution. Its architecture, a symphony of bone and ligament, is the underlying structure upon which the rich tapestry of human movement and feeling unfolds. Within the lumbar area of this mighty structure sits the lumbar epidural space, a sanctuary of possibility tucked between the vertebrae, awaiting the skillful touch of the anesthesiologist's hand.The spinal column, or vertebral column, is the primary axis of the human skeleton, giving structural support and protection to the fragile neural structures that lay therein. Composed of a series of stacked vertebrae, each bearing distinct anatomical characteristics and functions, the spinal column acts as the conduit via which critical information is conveyed between the brain and the rest of the body.At its cranial extremities sits the atlas, the first cervical vertebra, which cradles the head and enables for the essential action of nodding. Immediately underneath it, the axis, or second cervical vertebra, permits the rotation of the head, permitting the complicated dance of sensory perception and motor control.Descending farther up the spinal column, one finds the thoracic vertebrae, twelve in number, which engage with the ribs to create the thoracic cage, a protective enclosure for the essential organs of the chest cavity. Each thoracic vertebra possesses a pair of costal facets, which act as articulation sites for the ribs, maintaining the stability and movement of the thoracic spine.

Beyond the thoracic area is the lumbar spine, a region of special interest to lumbar epidural anesthesia. Comprising five vertebrae—designated L1 through L5—the lumbar spine bears the brunt of the body's weight and permits a broad variety of activities, from bending and lifting to walking and sprinting. The lumbar vertebrae are distinguished by their strong bodies and stout processes, which provide anchoring for the muscles and ligaments that support the spine.Between each pair of neighboring vertebrae sits an intervertebral disc, a fibrocartilaginous substance that functions as a cushion and shock absorber, allowing for smooth and pain-free movement of the spine. Composed of a gel-like nucleus pulposus surrounded by a strong annulus fibrosus, the intervertebral disc is well-adapted to endure the compression stresses put upon the spine during weight-bearing activities.The lumbar area of the spinal column is further differentiated by the presence of big, weight-bearing vertebral bodies and strong transverse processes, which offer attachment sites for the powerful muscles of the lower back. These muscles, comprising the erector spinae, multifidus, and quadratus lumborum, play a key role in maintaining and supporting the lumbar spine during movement and weight-bearing activities.

Of particular relevance to lumbar epidural anesthesia is the structure of the spinal canal, a hollow tube that contains the spinal cord and nerve roots. Bounded anteriorly by the vertebral bodies and posteriorly by the vertebral arches, the spinal canal acts as a protective channel for the neural tissues, safeguarding them from mechanical damage and external stress.Within the spinal canal sits the spinal cord, a cylindrical bundle of nerve fibers that stretches from the base of the brain to the level of the first lumbar vertebra. The spinal cord serves as the major channel for the transfer of sensory information from the peripheral nerves to the brain, as well as motor orders from the brain to the peripheral muscles and organs.Emerging from the spinal cord at regular intervals are pairs of spinal nerves, which leave the

CHAPTER 2

vertebral canal via tiny holes known as intervertebral foramina. These spinal nerves are important for transmitting sensory information from the periphery to the central nervous system, as well as motor orders from the central nervous system to the peripheral muscles and organs.Surrounding the spinal cord and nerve roots is a network of protective membranes known as the meninges, which help to cushion and feed the fragile neural tissues. The outermost layer of the meninges, known as the dura mater, is a thick and fibrous membrane that borders the inner wall of the vertebral canal, giving structural support and protection to the spinal cord and nerve roots.Beneath the dura mater is the arachnoid mater, a fragile membrane that forms a loose sheath over the spinal cord and nerve roots. Like a gossamer veil, the arachnoid mater acts as a barrier against infections and poisons, while allowing for the free flow of cerebrospinal fluid—a clear, colorless fluid that bathes and feeds the brain tissues.

Deep inside the depths of the spinal canal resides the pia mater, the deepest layer of the meninges that closely attaches to the surface of the spinal cord and nerve roots. Like a gentle hug, the pia mater gives sustenance and protection to the brain tissues, guaranteeing their well-being amongst the turbulent currents of life. It is this complicated network of structures—the spinal cord, nerve roots, and surrounding meninges—that creates the background against which lumbar epidural anesthesia develops.The lumbar epidural space, positioned between the dura mater and the bony spinal canal, indicates a potential region filled with adipose tissue and loose connective fibers. It is inside this anatomical domain that the magic of epidural anesthesia takes place, as the anesthesiologist navigates the needle through the surrounding tissues to enter the epidural region.Understanding the architecture of the lumbar spine and adjacent tissues is critical for the safe and successful administration of lumbar epidural anesthesia. Mastery of spinal anatomy helps the physician to recognize anatomical landmarks, determine the depth and direction of the epidural space, and reduce the danger of unintended harm to neural systems.

In essence, the lumbar spine is a wonder of biological engineering, encompassing a complicated network of bones, ligaments, nerves, and blood vessels. Within this complicated structure is the lumbar epidural area, a possible refuge for the delivery of epidural anesthesia. By having a complete grasp of spinal anatomy, doctors may assure the safe and successful administration of lumbar epidural anesthesia, affording patients respite from pain and suffering with confidence and accuracy.

2.2. Epidural Space Anatomy
Introduction

The use of lumbar epidural anesthesia is a cornerstone of current pain management and obstetric anesthetic procedures. This procedure, which includes the injection of local anesthetics or analgesics into the epidural region of the lumbar spine, offers excellent pain relief for a broad variety of therapeutic purposes, including labor analgesia, postoperative pain management, and chronic pain syndromes. However, the efficacy and safety of lumbar epidural anesthesia rest upon a detailed awareness of the anatomical structures and landmarks important to this technique.

In this chapter, we review the anatomy of the epidural space in depth, concentrating on its structure, regional variations, clinical consequences, and technical concerns for lumbar epidural anesthesia. By clarifying the numerous anatomical linkages within the lumbar spine, this chapter seeks to educate physicians with the information and skills essential to conduct lumbar epidural anesthesia safely and efficiently.

2.1 The Epidural Space: An Overview

The epidural space is a hypothetical anatomical compartment positioned between the dura mater and the bony spinal canal. It stretches longitudinally over the whole length of the spinal column, from the foramen magnum at the base of the skull to the sacral hiatus at the level of the sacrum. The epidural space is crossed by a network of blood arteries, adipose tissue, and connective tissue structures, which together regulate the accessibility and composition of the area.

2.1.1 Structure and Composition

The epidural space is defined by its distinctive shape and content, which play essential roles in determining the effectiveness and safety of epidural anesthetic delivery.

1. Dura Mater: The dura mater is the outermost layer of the meninges that wrap the spinal cord and contains the cerebrospinal fluid (CSF)-filled subarachnoid space. In the spinal column, the dura mater forms a tubular sheath known as the dural sac, which encases the spinal cord and stretches from the foramen magnum to the sacral hiatus.
2. Epidural Fat: Within the epidural space is adipose tissue, generally referred to as epidural fat. This adipose tissue offers cushioning and insulation for the spinal cord and nerve roots, helping to preserve these tissues from mechanical stress and damage. The distribution and density of epidural fat varies across people and throughout the spinal column, altering the depth and accessibility of the epidural space during anesthetic operations.
3. Spinal Ligaments: Surrounding the epidural space are different spinal ligaments, including the ligamentum flavum, anterior and posterior longitudinal ligaments, and interspinous ligaments. These ligaments contribute to the structural integrity of the vertebral column and assist keep the dura mater in place, avoiding excessive movement and displacement during spinal motion.

2.1.2 Regional Variations and Clinical Implications

The structure of the epidural space reveals regional differences throughout the spinal column, each having specific clinical consequences for lumbar epidural anesthetic techniques.

1. Thoracic Epidural Space: In the thoracic area, the epidural space is comparatively small and filled with a greater density of epidural fat compared to the lumbar region. As a consequence, thoracic epidural

anesthesia may need specific procedures to guarantee correct catheter insertion and maximal analgesic impact. Clinicians must care for these anatomical distinctions while conducting thoracic epidural operations to prevent unintended dural puncture or insufficient analgesia.

2. Lumbar Epidural Space: The lumbar epidural space, positioned between the vertebral lamina and the ligamentum flavum, is broader and more accessible compared to other parts of the spine. This makes it an attractive place for delivering epidural anesthetic, especially for surgeries affecting the lower belly, pelvis, and lower extremities. Clinicians may often execute lumbar epidural treatments with more ease and success because of the favorable anatomical qualities of the lumbar spine.

2.2 Epidural Space Anatomy

An in-depth grasp of epidural space anatomy is crucial for practitioners providing lumbar epidural anesthesia. This section includes a thorough analysis of the anatomical structures and landmarks pertinent to lumbar epidural operations, including the spinal vertebral column, ligamentous structures, and surrounding soft tissues.

2.2.1 Spinal Vertebral Column

The spinal vertebral column, also known as the spinal column or backbone, acts as the structural underpinning of the human body and contains the spinal cord, nerve roots, and surrounding vascular systems. Composed of distinct vertebrae separated by intervertebral discs, the vertebral column offers protection and support for the spinal cord while allowing for a broad range of motion in several planes.

1. Vertebral Regions: The vertebral column is split into several regions, including the cervical, thoracic, lumbar, sacral, and coccygeal regions, each defined by distinctive anatomical traits and functional qualities. The lumbar spine, consisting of five vertebrae (L1-L5), comprises the

bottom region of the vertebral column and is of special significance to lumbar epidural anesthetic operations.
2. Intervertebral Foramina: Located between neighboring vertebrae are intervertebral foramina, which act as conduits for spinal nerves as they depart the spinal cord and travel to different areas of the body. The size and direction of the intervertebral foramina vary throughout the spinal column, impacting the trajectory of spinal needles and catheters during epidural treatments.

2.2.2 Ligamentous Structures

The epidural space is bordered by various ligamentous structures that offer stability and support to the spinal column while assisting to preserve the integrity of the epidural space.

1. Ligamentum Flavum: The ligamentum flavum, often known as the yellow ligament, is a thick, elastic ligament that crosses the posterior portion of the spinal canal. It joins the laminae of neighboring vertebrae and helps maintain the proper curvature of the spine. During lumbar epidural treatments, the ligamentum flavum acts as a significant anatomical reference for identifying the epidural area and directing needle entry.
2. Anterior and Posterior Longitudinal Ligaments: The anterior and posterior longitudinal ligaments run along the anterior and posterior surfaces of the vertebral bodies, respectively, giving extra support to the vertebral column. While the anterior longitudinal ligament largely inhibits excessive extension of the spine, the posterior longitudinal ligament helps resist hyperflexion and gives support to the intervertebral discs.
3. Supraspinous and Interspinous Ligaments: Located posteriorly throughout the vertebral column are the supraspinous and interspinous ligaments, which link the spinous processes of neighboring vertebrae. These ligaments assist maintain alignment and stability between

vertebral segments, functioning as attachment sites for muscles and providing resistance to excessive spinal flexion and extension.

2.2.3 Soft Tissues

In addition to bone and ligamentous components, the epidural space is bordered by numerous soft tissues, including adipose tissue, blood vessels, and nerve roots, which contribute to the overall composition and function of the epidural space.

1. Epidural Fat: Adipose tissue, generally referred to as epidural fat, inhabits the epidural space and functions as a protective cushion for the spinal cord and nerve roots. The distribution and density of epidural fat differ across people, altering the accessibility and depth of the epidural space during anesthetic operations. Clinicians must consider for changes in epidural fat content while conducting lumbar epidural treatments to ensure proper needle insertion and maximal analgesic impact.
2. Blood Vessels: The epidural space has a network of blood vessels, including arteries, veins, and capillaries, which deliver nutrition and oxygen to the surrounding tissues. These veins serve a key function in sustaining the circulatory supply to the spinal cord and nerve roots while also aiding the dispersion of administered drugs inside the epidural region.
3. Nerve Roots: Nerve roots arising from the spinal cord cross the epidural space as they leave the intervertebral foramina and proceed to their respective target tissues. These nerve roots are prone to compression or discomfort during epidural anesthetic operations, especially if the needle or catheter accidentally hits or enters the neural structures. Careful care must be taken to prevent nerve damage and decrease the risk of neurological problems during lumbar epidural treatments.

CHAPTER 2

2.3 Clinical Considerations and Techniques

Performing lumbar epidural anesthesia needs a mix of anatomical understanding, technical expertise, and clinical judgment. Clinicians must apply suitable procedures and procedural considerations to guarantee the safety and effectiveness of epidural anesthetic treatment.

2.3.1 Patient Positioning

Proper patient posture is critical for aiding successful needle insertion and catheter advancement during lumbar epidural treatments. The patient is often positioned in either the sitting or lateral decubitus position, depending on the clinical circumstance and the discretion of the anesthetic practitioner.

1. Sitting Position: In the sitting position, the patient sits erect on the edge of the operating table with their back flexed and their legs hanging over the side. This posture provides for gravity-assisted descent of the spinal cord and enlargement of the intervertebral gaps, permitting better needle insertion and access to the epidural area.
2. Lateral Decubitus Position: Alternatively, the patient may be positioned in the lateral decubitus position, laying on their side with their back aligned parallel to the edge of the operating table. This posture enables lateral access to the lumbar spine and allows for accurate identification of vertebral landmarks and needle insertion locations.

2.3.2 Needle Insertion Techniques

The method utilized for needle insertion during lumbar epidural anesthesia varies based on the clinical reason, patient features, and provider choice. Common ways include the midline and paramedian procedures, each with its own benefits and concerns.

1. Midline technique: The midline technique includes placing the needle down the midline of the patient's back, aiming the interspinous area between neighboring spinous processes. This method allows direct

access to the midline epidural space and is commonly utilized for regular epidural treatments in the lumbar area. Palpation of bone landmarks and cautious advancement of the needle under fluoroscopy or ultrasound guidance assure proper insertion inside the epidural space.
2. Paramedian method: Alternatively, the paramedian method comprises putting the needle lateral to the midline, targeting the epidural area close to the spinous process. This procedure may be preferable in individuals with spinal abnormalities, obesity, or anatomical differences that make the midline approach hard. Ultrasound or fluoroscopic assistance may help in seeing the target region and directing needle insertion, boosting the precision and safety of the paramedian approach.

2.3.3 Catheter Advancement and Medication Administration

Once the epidural area is reached successfully, a flexible catheter is often pushed through the needle into the epidural space to permit continuous drug administration. Local anesthetics, analgesics, or combination solutions may be delivered via the epidural catheter to offer pain relief, anesthesia, or both, depending on the clinical reason and patient demands.

1. Catheter location: After verifying the intravascular or intrathecal location of the needle, the catheter is put through the needle into the epidural area and held in place using an adhesive dressing or suture. Careful care must be taken to prevent catheter movement or dislodgement, which may affect drug administration and effectiveness.
2. Drug Selection and dose: The choice of drug and dose regimen relies on several criteria, including the patient's medical history, pain intensity, and procedural needs. Clinicians must follow established criteria and safety measures while choosing and delivering epidural drugs to reduce the risk of adverse events and maintain patient comfort and safety.

2.4 Complications and Risk Mitigation

Despite precise skill and attention to safety measures, lumbar epidural anesthetic techniques entail intrinsic risks of complications, including dural puncture, nerve damage, hematoma development, and infection. Clinicians must be diligent in recognizing and treating these problems to promote optimum patient outcomes and reduce morbidity and death.

2.4.1 Dural Puncture

Accidental dural puncture, or "wet tap," happens when the epidural needle unintentionally breaks the dura mater, resulting in leaking of cerebrospinal fluid (CSF) into the epidural space. Dural puncture is a moderately frequent complication of lumbar epidural treatments, occurring in up to 1-2% of instances.

1. Clinical Presentation: Patients who undergo dural puncture may develop symptoms of post-dural puncture headache (PDPH), including frontal or occipital headache, neck stiffness, nausea, and photophobia. The intensity and duration of symptoms varies based on the degree of CSF leaking and specific patient characteristics.
2. Management Strategies: Management of dural puncture encompasses conservative approaches to ease symptoms and encourage CSF re-absorption, as well as interventional procedures such as epidural blood patching to seal the dural defect and restore CSF pressure. Close monitoring and follow-up are important to assure remission of symptoms and avoid consequences.

2.4.2 Nerve Injury

Nerve damage is an uncommon but potentially dangerous consequence of lumbar epidural anesthesia, arising from direct trauma, compression, or ischemia of neural structures inside the epidural space. Nerve damage may appear as sensory or motor impairments, radicular discomfort, or autonomic dysfunction, depending on the location and degree of the lesion.

1. Risk risks: Risk risks for nerve damage include needle trauma, catheter insertion, high injection pressures, and pre-existing neurological disorders. Patient characteristics such as age, body habitus, and anatomical variances may potentially increase the chance of nerve damage during epidural treatments.
2. Prevention and Management: Prevention of nerve damage needs rigorous technique, cautious patient selection, and suitable needle and catheter insertion under direct visualization or imaging guidance. Early diagnosis and timely therapy of neurological symptoms are critical to decrease the risk of long-term consequences and enhance patient outcomes.

2.4.3 Hematoma Formation

Hematoma development inside the epidural space is an uncommon but potentially life-threatening consequence of lumbar epidural anesthesia, especially in patients undergoing anticoagulant or antiplatelet treatment. Epidural hematomas may compress neuronal tissues inside the spinal canal, leading to neurological impairments and spinal cord damage.

- Clinical Presentation: Patients with epidural hematomas may present with signs of spinal cord compression, including back discomfort, sensory impairments, motor weakness, and bowel or bladder dysfunction. Prompt identification and treatments are crucial to avoid lasting neurological injury and maintain spinal function.

Risk Mitigation and Management

Mitigating the risk of hematoma development entails thorough patient evaluation, pre-procedural screening for bleeding disorders or coagulopathies, and cautious administration of anticoagulant and antiplatelet drugs. In patients with known bleeding diathesis or high-risk thromboembolic disorders, alternate analgesic approaches or adjustments to anticoagulation regimes may be explored to limit the risk of hematoma development.

1. Management Strategies: Management of epidural hematomas needs prompt detection and urgent action to decompress the spinal cord and avoid irreparable neurological impairment. Surgical evacuation of the hematoma may be indicated in situations of substantial spinal cord compression or developing neurological impairments. Close coordination between anesthetic physicians, neurosurgeons, and hematologists is crucial to enhance patient outcomes and decrease morbidity and mortality associated with epidural hematomas.

2.4.4 Infection

Infection is an uncommon but potentially significant consequence of lumbar epidural anesthesia, with the potential to induce epidural abscesses, meningitis, or systemic sepsis. Risk factors for epidural infection include contaminated equipment, incorrect aseptic technique, extended catheter dwell periods, and underlying immunocompromised conditions.

1. Clinical Presentation: Patients with epidural infections may show with localized discomfort, erythema, edema, or discharge at the site of needle insertion, as well as systemic indications of infection such as fever, chills, and malaise. Prompt identification and early beginning of antibiotic treatment are critical to minimize the spread of infection and decrease the risk of systemic consequences.
2. Prevention Strategies: Prevention of epidural infections involves rigorous attention to aseptic technique, including thorough hand cleanliness, skin preparation, and sterile draping during lumbar epidural treatments. Regular monitoring of catheter insertion sites and early removal of catheters when no longer necessary will help limit the incidence of catheter-related infections. Additionally, prudent administration of prophylactic antibiotics may be explored in high-risk patients receiving extended epidural anesthesia or those with pre-

existing comorbidities predisposing them to infection.

2.5 Conclusion

Lumbar epidural anesthesia is a powerful weapon in the armamentarium of pain management and anesthesia procedures, giving excellent pain reduction and anesthesia for a broad variety of therapeutic causes. However, the effectiveness and safety of epidural anesthetic operations rest upon a complete grasp of epidural space anatomy, excellent technique, and watchful attention to possible issues.By fully addressing the anatomical features, regional variations, clinical consequences, and procedural concerns pertinent to lumbar epidural anesthesia, practitioners may strengthen their expertise and confidence in executing these operations. Adherence to established protocols, continued education, and multidisciplinary teamwork are critical for enhancing patient outcomes and limiting the risk of problems associated with lumbar epidural anesthesia.

In conclusion, lumbar epidural anesthesia is a cornerstone of contemporary anesthesia treatment, giving safe and effective pain management for patients undergoing a broad variety of surgical and obstetric procedures. By learning the anatomy of the epidural space and utilizing suitable procedures and precautions, doctors may assure the effective administration of epidural anesthesia while reducing the risk of problems and boosting patient comfort and satisfaction.

2.3 Neurovascular Structures: Navigating the Complex Pathways

In the area of lumbar epidural anesthesia, the comprehension of neurovascular systems running through the epidural region is not just advantageous; it's vital. This section goes on an extensive trip through the anatomical paths of nerves and blood vessels, emphasizing their relevance in the administration and safety of epidural anesthesia.

2.3.1 Nerves: Pathways of Sensation and Motor Function

CHAPTER 2

Nerves are the conduits of sensation and motor function, delicately interlaced into the fabric of the epidural region. Understanding their trajectories and distributions is critical for the exact administration of anesthetic and analgesia.

1. Spinal Nerves: Emerging from the intervertebral foramina, spinal nerves cross the epidural space en route to their peripheral destinations. These nerves deliver sensory information from the body to the spinal cord (afferent fibers) and transfer motor orders from the spinal cord to the muscles (efferent fibers).
2. Dermatomes and Myotomes: Each spinal neuron innervates a particular area of the body known as a dermatome, responsible for sensory perception. Additionally, spinal nerves relate to particular muscle groups known as myotomes, directing motor performance. Clinicians must possess a comprehensive grasp of dermatome and myotome anatomy to adapt epidural anesthesia to specific patient requirements efficiently.
3. Differences and Clinical Correlations: Anatomical differences in nerve distribution and innervation patterns may impact the choice of epidural method and the dissemination of anesthesia. Moreover, correlations between dermatomal distribution and clinical symptoms play a key role in detecting and controlling pain disorders, such as radiculopathy and neuropathy.

2.3.2 Vasculature: Rivers of Life

The vasculature of the epidural space functions as the lifeblood, feeding neural structures and guaranteeing their viability. A grasp of vascular architecture is crucial for minimizing the risk of hemorrhagic consequences during epidural treatments.

1. Arteries and Veins: Arteries carry oxygenated blood to the spinal cord and associated neural structures, while veins assist the return of

deoxygenated blood to the systemic circulation. The delicate balance between arterial input and venous outflow must be managed to ensure proper tissue perfusion and avoid ischemic damage.
2. Venous Plexus: Within the epidural space is a network of veins known as the epidural venous plexus, which drains blood from the vertebral column and spinal cord. The epidural venous plexus is especially prone to engorgement and bleeding during epidural needle insertion, underlining the significance of rigorous technique and anatomical awareness.
3. Collateral Circulation: The existence of collateral circulation inside the epidural space offers an alternate conduit for blood flow in the case of arterial impairment or obstruction. Clinicians must be conscious of collateral vessels and their potential to ameliorate the consequences of vascular insufficiency during epidural operations.

2.3.3 Clinical Implications: Navigating the Neurovascular Maze

The complicated interaction between neurovascular systems provides both obstacles and possibilities in the domain of lumbar epidural anesthesia. Clinicians must negotiate this complicated terrain with accuracy and elegance to enhance patient outcomes and limit the risk of consequences.

1. Safety Considerations: The closeness of nerves and blood vessels inside the epidural region needs a careful approach to needle insertion and catheter advancement. Clinicians must exert caution to minimize unintended neurological or vascular harm, leveraging imaging guidance and anatomical landmarks to increase procedural precision.
2. Complication Management: Despite rigorous technique, problems such as hematoma development, nerve damage, and vascular trauma may emerge during lumbar epidural treatments. Prompt detection and action are critical to decrease the severity of problems and ensure patient well-being. Collaboration with multidisciplinary teams, including neurologists, vascular surgeons, and hematologists, may be

important to manage complicated issues efficiently.
3. Risk Stratification: Pre-procedural evaluation and risk stratification are critical stages in guaranteeing the safety and effectiveness of lumbar epidural anesthesia. Clinicians must analyze patient-specific characteristics, including coagulation status, medication usage, and anatomical considerations, to identify patients at higher risk of problems and modify anesthetic therapy appropriately.

2.3.4 Technical Considerations: Mastering the Art of Precision

Achieving expertise in lumbar epidural anesthesia involves more than just theoretical understanding; it demands technical skill and procedural delicacy. Clinicians must enhance their abilities in needle insertion, catheter advancement, and medicine administration to maximize patient comfort and safety.

1. Needle Placement: The method utilized for needle insertion during lumbar epidural anesthesia varies based on the clinical reason, patient characteristics, and provider choice. Common ways include the midline and paramedian procedures, each with its own benefits and concerns.
2. Catheter Advancement: Once the epidural space is reached successfully, a flexible catheter is routinely advanced through the needle into the epidural area to provide continuous drug administration. Careful care must be taken to ensure correct catheter insertion and attachment to avoid displacement or migration.
3. Drug Selection and dose: The choice of drug and dose regimen relies on several criteria, including the patient's medical history, pain intensity, and procedural needs. Clinicians must follow established criteria and safety measures while choosing and delivering epidural drugs to reduce the risk of adverse events and maintain patient comfort and safety.

Conclusion: Navigating the Anatomical Maze with Precision and Skill

In the labyrinthine environment of lumbar epidural anesthesia, a full grasp of neurovascular systems is the compass that directs practitioners toward safe and successful patient management. By knowing the subtleties of nerve and vascular anatomy, doctors may traverse the epidural region with precision and competence, maximizing anesthetic administration and lowering the risk of complications. In this complicated dance of anatomy and technique, knowledge is the key to unlocking success, and competence is the hand that directs us toward calmer beaches.

Chapter 3

PHYSIOLOGY OF EPIDURAL ANESTHESIA

3.1 Mechanism of Action: Unraveling the Intricacies

In the fabric of pain management, epidural anesthesia stands as a masterpiece, giving significant comfort via its complicated mechanisms of action. This chapter dives into the physiological basis of epidural anesthesia, revealing the complexity of its process and offering light on its therapeutic usefulness.

3.1.1 The Epidural Space: Gateway to Relief

At the core of epidural anesthesia lies the epidural space, a hypothetical anatomical compartment positioned between the dura mater and the bony spinal canal. This region acts as the gateway for the introduction of local anesthetics or analgesics, which exert their effects on the spinal cord and adjacent neuronal structures to cause pain relief and anesthesia.

3.1.2 Mechanisms of Local Anesthetic Action

Local anesthetics, the cornerstone of epidural anesthesia, exert their effects by preventing the formation and propagation of action potentials in peripheral nerves. This blocking occurs via the inhibition of voltage-gated sodium channels, which are important for the fast depolarization and propagation of nerve impulses.

1. Binding and Inactivation: Upon injection into the epidural space, local anesthetics bind to voltage-gated sodium channels present on the axonal membrane of peripheral neurons. This binding restricts the entrance of sodium ions, hence suppressing depolarization and preventing the formation of action potentials.
2. Differential Sensitivity: Not all nerve fibers are equally responsive to local anesthetic inhibition. Small, unmyelinated C fibers, responsible for conveying sluggish, dull pain sensations, are more vulnerable to local anesthetic blocking compared to bigger, myelinated A fibers, which transmit intense, quick pain sensations. This selective blockage allows for distinct regulation of pain perception dependent on fiber type and diameter.

3.1.3 Spread of Epidural Anesthesia

The distribution of epidural anesthesia inside the epidural space is regulated by numerous variables, including the amount and concentration of local anesthetic administered, patient positioning, and anatomical considerations. Understanding the factors of epidural distribution is critical for personalizing anesthetic to specific patient demands and enhancing clinical results.

1. Gravity and placement: Patient placement has a key role in regulating the distribution and amount of epidural anesthetic dissemination. In the upright posture, gravity increases caudal migration of local anesthetic inside the epidural space, resulting in more comprehensive coverage of lower dermatomes. Conversely, in the supine or lateral posture, gravity has less impact on epidural dissemination, resulting in more localized anesthetic distribution.
2. Volume and Concentration: The volume and concentration of local anesthetic injected into the spinal region directly impact the amount and duration of anesthesia. Larger quantities of dilute solutions result in wider anesthetic dissemination but may be linked with higher risk of

systemic toxicity. Conversely, lesser amounts of concentrated solutions generate more localized anesthetic but may offer inadequate coverage for prolonged surgical operations.

3.1.4 Modulation of Pain Transmission

Beyond its function in inhibiting nerve conduction, epidural anesthesia regulates pain transmission via intricate interactions with neurotransmitter systems inside the spinal cord. By modifying the release and absorption of neurotransmitters, epidural anesthesia has dramatic effects on pain perception and processing, giving both analgesic and antinociceptive advantages.

1. GABAergic Inhibition: Local anesthetics boost gamma-aminobutyric acid (GABA)-mediated inhibitory neurotransmission inside the spinal cord, resulting in hyperpolarization of postsynaptic neurons and attenuation of pain signals. This GABAergic inhibition lowers neuronal excitability and dampens nociceptive transmission, leading to the analgesic benefits of epidural anesthesia.
2. NMDA Receptor Blockade: In addition to GABAergic modulation, local anesthetics oppose N-methyl-D-aspartate (NMDA) receptors inside the spinal cord, reducing excitatory neurotransmission and avoiding central sensitization. By preventing the activation of NMDA receptors, epidural anesthesia lowers the amplification of pain signals and inhibits the development of chronic pain states.

3.1.5 Autonomic Effects of Epidural Anesthesia

Epidural anesthesia produces substantial effects on the autonomic nervous system, altering cardiovascular, respiratory, and gastrointestinal function. These autonomic effects are mediated by interactions with sympathetic and parasympathetic circuits within the spinal cord, resulting in variations in physiological balance and systemic hemodynamics.

1. **Sympathetic Blockade:** Epidural anesthesia generates sympathetic blockade by limiting the passage of sympathetic efferent impulses from the spinal cord to peripheral organs. This blockage leads to vasodilation, hypotension, and bradycardia, as well as abnormalities in thermoregulation and sweating patterns.
2. **Parasympathetic Modulation:** In addition to sympathetic blocking, epidural anesthesia affects parasympathetic tone via its effects on preganglionic parasympathetic neurons inside the spinal cord. This modulation leads to variations in gastrointestinal motility, bladder function, and bronchial tone, altering total visceral homeostasis.

3.1.6 Duration and Recovery of Epidural Anesthesia

The duration and recovery of epidural anesthesia are regulated by a variety of variables, including the pharmacokinetics of the local anesthetic agent, the volume and concentration of the epidural solution, patient characteristics, and the presence of supplementary drugs. Understanding the dynamics of epidural anesthetic duration and recovery is critical for improving patient care and limiting the risk of adverse events.

1. **Pharmacokinetics:** The pharmacokinetic features of local anesthetics govern their start, duration, and offset of action inside the epidural area. Factors such as lipid solubility, protein binding, and metabolism impact the pace of local anesthetic absorption, distribution, and elimination, eventually influencing the duration of epidural anesthesia effects.
2. **Volume and Concentration:** The volume and concentration of the epidural solution play a key role in influencing the duration and degree of anesthesia. Higher volumes of local anesthetic result in more comprehensive neuronal blockage and longer duration of action, but higher concentrations generate more rapid onset and shorter duration of anesthesia.
3. **Patient Characteristics:** Individual patient characteristics, such as age, weight, comorbidities, and concomitant drugs, might alter the

pharmacokinetics and pharmacodynamics of epidural anesthesia. Elderly individuals and those with poor hepatic or renal function may display longer duration of anesthesia owing to impaired drug clearance, while obese patients may need greater dosages of local anesthetic to get acceptable pain relief.
4. Adjunctive drugs: The addition of adjunctive drugs, such as opioids, adjuvants, or vasoconstrictors, to the epidural solution may alter the duration and quality of anesthesia. Opioids increase the duration of analgesia by acting on opioid receptors inside the spinal cord, while adjuvants such as epinephrine improve the distribution and duration of local anesthetic blockade via vasoconstrictive actions.

3.1.7 Clinical Applications and Considerations

Understanding the mechanism of action of epidural anesthesia is crucial for its safe and successful usage across many clinical situations. From perioperative pain management to obstetric analgesia, epidural anesthesia provides various applications that may be adjusted to particular patient demands and procedural restrictions.

1. Perioperative Pain Management: Epidural anesthesia plays a crucial role in multimodal analgesia techniques for perioperative pain management, delivering greater pain reduction compared to systemic opioids alone. By delivering focused analgesia and limiting opioid needs, epidural anesthesia minimizes postoperative pain severity, opioid-related adverse effects, and duration of hospital stay.
2. Obstetric Analgesia: Epidural anesthesia is the cornerstone of labor analgesia, providing adequate pain relief while maintaining mother motor function and allowing instrumental births. Continuous epidural infusion methods allow for adjustment of anesthetic depth and duration, enabling optimum pain management throughout the phases of labor and delivery.
3. Chronic Pain Management: In the field of chronic pain management,

epidural anesthesia acts as a significant treatment tool for illnesses such as lumbar radiculopathy, spinal stenosis, and complicated regional pain syndrome. Epidural steroid injections, paired with local anesthetics, give focused anti-inflammatory effects and neuronal blocking, offering long-lasting pain relief and functional improvement.

3.1.8 Safety Considerations and Complications

While epidural anesthesia provides substantial advantages in pain control and anesthesia, it is not without dangers. Complications linked with epidural anesthesia include hematoma development, nerve damage, infection, and systemic toxicity, which may come from needle trauma, catheter misplacement, or medication-related side effects.

1. Hematoma development: Epidural hematoma development, however uncommon, offers a substantial danger of spinal cord compression and neurological damage. Clinicians must adhere to rigorous aseptic technique, monitor coagulation status, and undertake neurologic tests to identify early indicators of hematoma development and act swiftly.
2. Nerve damage: Nerve damage resulting from direct trauma or compression inside the epidural space may lead to sensory or motor impairments, neuropathic pain, or autonomic dysfunction. Careful needle insertion, avoidance of excessive force during catheter advancement, and periodic neurologic monitoring are crucial for limiting the risk of nerve damage.
3. Infection: Epidural infection, albeit rare, may result in epidural abscess, meningitis, or sepsis, presenting considerable morbidity and mortality concerns. Strict attention to aseptic procedures, careful skin preparation, and frequent catheter site examination are critical for avoiding infection and lowering the risk of systemic consequences.
4. Systemic Toxicity: Systemic toxicity from local anesthetic absorption may occur if large dosages are provided or if the epidural solution mistakenly reaches the systemic circulation. Early detection of systemic

toxicity symptoms, such as seizures, cardiovascular collapse, or central nervous system depression, is crucial for commencing fast therapy and averting catastrophic consequences.

Conclusion: Mastering the Art and Science of Epidural Anesthesia

In the complicated dance of physiology and pharmacology, epidural anesthesia emerges as a beacon of hope, delivering significant respite from pain and suffering. By uncovering the mechanisms of action, understanding the intricacies of drug dynamics, and adopting the principles of patient-centered care, doctors may harness the full potential of epidural anesthesia to maximize patient outcomes and increase quality of life. In our quest of perfection, knowledge is our compass, skill is our guide, and compassion is our driving force.

3.2: Pharmacokinetics and Pharmacodynamics

In the area of anesthesia, knowing the pharmacokinetics and pharmacodynamics of epidural anesthesia is crucial. This section dives into the delicate interaction between drug kinetics and dynamics, elucidating the mechanics underlying the onset, duration, and consequences of epidural anesthesia.

Pharmacokinetics: Understanding the Journey of the Drug

Pharmacokinetics involves the absorption, distribution, metabolism, and excretion (ADME) of pharmaceuticals inside the body. In the context of epidural anesthesia, pharmacokinetics elucidates how local anesthetic drugs transit biological barriers, interact with tissues, and are finally eliminated from the body.

1. Absorption: Following epidural administration, local anesthetics penetrate the epidural space to reach their target locations inside the spinal cord and peripheral nerves. Factors such as medication concentration, lipid solubility, and tissue vascularity impact the pace

and amount of drug absorption. Lipophilic drugs tend to diffuse more rapidly across cell membranes, whereas highly perfused tissues enable fast drug equilibration.
2. Distribution: Once absorbed, local anesthetics diffuse throughout the epidural space and neighboring neural tissues, attaching to protein receptors and exerting their pharmacological effects. Distribution is determined by variables such as tissue perfusion, protein binding affinity, and regional blood flow. Highly perfused tissues such as the spinal cord and nerve roots acquire larger amounts of local anesthetics compared to less vascularized tissues.
3. Metabolism: Local anesthetics undergo biotransformation in the liver and other organs, largely via hepatic cytochrome P450 enzymes. Metabolic pathways vary across various local anesthetic drugs, creating metabolites that are either pharmacologically active or inert. The rate of metabolism determines drug clearance and duration of action, with slower metabolism resulting in extended pharmacological effects.
4. Excretion: Metabolites of local anesthetics are removed from the body by renal excretion, with urine clearance playing a substantial role in drug removal. Renal impairment may impede medication clearance and lengthen drug half-life, requiring dose modifications in individuals with renal failure. In addition to renal excretion, local anesthetics may undergo biliary excretion or undergo enterohepatic recycling, further affecting their pharmacokinetic profile.

3.2.1 Pharmacodynamics: Unraveling the Mechanisms of Action

Pharmacodynamics elucidates how medications interact with biological targets to elicit physiological effects. In the instance of epidural anesthesia, pharmacodynamics elucidates how local anesthetics regulate neuronal excitability, suppress nociceptive signals, and produce sensory and motor blocking.

1. blocking of Nerve Conduction: The principal pharmacodynamic

action of local anesthetics is the blocking of voltage-gated sodium channels in peripheral nerves. By binding to particular receptor sites on sodium channels, local anesthetics limit the inflow of sodium ions, inhibiting depolarization and propagation of action potentials. This blockade is reversible and dose-dependent, with larger drug concentrations resulting in more severe brain blockage.
2. Modulation of Pain Perception: In addition to their effects on nerve conduction, local anesthetics affect pain perception by modulating neurotransmitter release and synaptic transmission within the spinal cord. By boosting inhibitory neurotransmission and reducing excitatory neurotransmission, local anesthetics reduce nociceptive signals and decrease pain experience. This modulation happens largely in the dorsal horn of the spinal cord, where primary afferent fibers synapse with second-order neurons implicated in pain processing.
3. Sensory and Motor Blockade: Epidural anesthesia creates sensory and motor blockade by selectively suppressing the transmission of sensory and motor impulses inside the spinal cord. Sensory blockage results in loss of pain feeling and temperature awareness, while motor blockade leads to muscular weakening and paralysis. The amount and duration of blocking depend on parameters such as drug concentration, volume, and dispersion within the epidural space.

3.2.2 Clinical Implications and Considerations

Understanding the pharmacokinetic and pharmacodynamic aspects of epidural anesthesia is critical for enhancing patient care and assuring safe and efficient anesthesia administration. Clinicians must examine several criteria, including patient characteristics, medication selection, dosage regimens, and monitoring measures, to obtain optimum results and limit the risk of adverse events.

1. Patient Characteristics: Individual patient parameters such as age, weight, comorbidities, and concomitant drugs might alter the phar-

macokinetics and pharmacodynamics of epidural anesthesia. Elderly individuals may demonstrate altered drug metabolism and clearance, whereas obese people may need greater doses to induce sufficient anesthesia. Careful patient evaluation and tailored treatment strategies are crucial for adapting anesthetic regimens to each patient's requirements.

2. Drug Selection & Dosing: The choice of local anesthetic agent, concentration, and volume for epidural anesthesia relies on parameters such as the desired depth and duration of anesthesia, the kind of surgical operation, and the patient's clinical status. brief-acting drugs such as lidocaine are useful for treatments requiring quick onset and brief duration of anesthetic, whereas long-acting medicines such as bupivacaine and ropivacaine are chosen for extended pain relief and postoperative analgesia. Dosing regimens should be based on patient weight, age, and comorbidities, with careful attention given to maximum suggested dosages and toxicity thresholds.

3. Monitoring and Management: Continuous monitoring of vital signs, neurological condition, and medication effects is important during epidural anesthetic administration. Regular examinations of sensory and motor function, hemodynamic stability, and respiratory state enable early diagnosis of problems such as local anesthetic toxicity, nerve damage, or hemodynamic instability. Prompt action and proper treatment measures, including medication reversal, supportive care, and escalation of care if required, are critical for decreasing the risk of adverse events and preserving patient safety.

Conclusion: Harnessing the Power of Pharmacology in Epidural Anesthesia

In the complicated terrain of epidural anesthesia, pharmacokinetics and pharmacodynamics serve as guiding principles for safe and efficient anesthetic administration. By knowing the route of the medication inside the body and uncovering the processes underlying its pharmacological effects, doctors may traverse the complexities of epidural anesthesia with accuracy and confidence. Through rigorous patient evaluation, intelligent medication selection, and diligent monitoring, epidural anesthesia may be used as a potent instrument for pain management and anesthesia, improving patient outcomes and boosting the quality of treatment.

3.3 Effects on the Nervous System: Navigating the Neural Terrain

In the complicated dance between pharmacology and physiology, the effects of epidural anesthesia on the nervous system emerge with precision and intricacy. This chapter goes on a tour across the neural landscape, studying how epidural anesthesia impacts sensory perception, motor function, and autonomic reactions.

Unraveling Sensory Modulation

Epidural anesthesia has dramatic effects on sensory processing inside the central nervous system, affecting the experience of pain and sensory inputs. By specifically targeting nociceptive pathways, epidural anesthesia offers excellent analgesia and pain reduction, boosting patient comfort during surgical operations and after recovery.

1. Sensory blockage: The characteristic of epidural anesthesia is sensory blockage, which limits the passage of pain signals from peripheral nerves to the spinal cord and brain. Local anesthetics injected into the epidural space diffuse to the dorsal horn of the spinal cord, where they interact with sensory neurons and suppress nociceptive signals. This blocking leads to loss of feeling and pain perception in the dermatomal distribution corresponding to the level of epidural catheter implantation.
2. Modulation of Pain Perception: Beyond just blocking pain signals, epidural anesthesia affects pain perception by modifying synaptic transmission and neurotransmitter release inside the spinal cord. By boosting inhibitory neurotransmission mediated by gamma-aminobutyric acid (GABA) and glycine receptors, while decreasing excitatory neurotransmission mediated by glutamate receptors, epidural anesthesia

effectively dampens nociceptive signals and lowers the subjective perception of pain.
3. Segmental Anesthesia: Epidural anesthesia induces segmental anesthesia, meaning that sensory blockage is restricted to particular dermatomes innervated by the spinal nerves next to the site of epidural injection. The amount and intensity of sensory blocking rely on parameters such as the volume and concentration of local anesthetic administered, the diffusion of drugs inside the epidural region, and individual patient characteristics.

Navigating Motor Inhibition

In addition to sensory effects, epidural anesthesia may also elicit motor blockage, decreasing voluntary muscle activity and motor coordination. By targeting motor pathways inside the spinal cord, epidural anesthetic produces muscular weakness and paralysis, enabling surgical access and limiting patient movement during operations.

1. Motor Blockade: Epidural anesthesia limits motor function by preventing the passage of motor impulses from the spinal cord to peripheral muscles. Local anesthetics injected into the epidural space diffuse to the ventral horn of the spinal cord, where they interact with motor neurons and interfere with neuromuscular transmission. This blocking leads to muscular weakness and paralysis in the myotomal distribution corresponding to the level of epidural catheter implantation.
2. Dose-Dependent Effects: The degree of motor blockage generated by epidural anesthesia is dose-dependent, with larger doses of local anesthetic resulting in more severe muscle weakening. Clinicians may vary the dosage and concentration of local anesthetic to obtain the necessary amount of motor blockade for certain surgical procedures, balancing the necessity for surgical access with the preservation of motor function in non-operative muscle groups.
3. Selective Muscle Relaxation: Epidural anesthesia may be modified

to generate selective muscle relaxation, enabling surgeons to target particular muscle groups while maintaining motor function in others. By modifying the amount and distribution of local anesthetic inside the epidural space, doctors may accomplish differential blocking of motor neurons innervating distinct muscle groups, enhancing surgical circumstances and patient comfort.

Balancing Autonomic Modulation

Epidural anesthesia has profound effects on the autonomic nervous system, altering cardiovascular, respiratory, and gastrointestinal function. By modifying sympathetic and parasympathetic tone within the spinal cord, epidural anesthesia may elicit substantial changes in vital signs, blood flow, and organ function, demanding careful monitoring and control throughout anesthetic delivery.

1. Sympathetic Blockade: Epidural anesthesia generates sympathetic blockade by reducing sympathetic outflow from the spinal cord, resulting in vasodilation, hypotension, and bradycardia. By preventing the transmission of sympathetic impulses to peripheral blood vessels and the heart, epidural anesthesia decreases systemic vascular resistance and cardiac output, resulting in lowered blood pressure and heart rate.
2. Hemodynamic Stability: The hemodynamic effects of epidural anesthesia may be severe, especially in individuals with reduced cardiovascular function or pre-existing autonomic dysfunction. Clinicians must monitor vital signs regularly during epidural anesthetic administration, predicting and controlling hemodynamic changes rapidly to avoid hypotension, arrhythmias, or other cardiovascular problems.
3. Respiratory Effects: Epidural anesthesia may also impair respiratory function by affecting diaphragmatic excursion, respiratory muscle strength, and ventilatory drive. While epidural anesthesia normally preserves respiratory function, severe degrees of sensory blockage or simultaneous administration of sedative medicines might impede

respiratory effort and raise the risk of hypoventilation or respiratory compromise.
4. Gastrointestinal Effects: Epidural anesthesia may alter gastrointestinal motility and function by changing autonomic inputs to the gastrointestinal tract. Sympathetic blockade may result in reduced gastrointestinal tone and motility, leading to delayed gastric emptying, ileus, or constipation. Clinicians must evaluate bowel function regularly during epidural anesthetic administration, employing strategies to avoid or treat gastrointestinal problems.

Conclusion: Navigating the Neurological Terrain of Epidural Anesthesia

In the delicate interaction between pharmacology and physiology, epidural anesthesia has dramatic effects on the nervous system, modifying sensory perception, motor function, and autonomic responses. By understanding the processes behind these effects, doctors may improve anesthetic distribution, limit problems, and increase patient safety and comfort during surgical operations. Through rigorous monitoring and treatment of neurological parameters, epidural anesthesia may be used as a potent instrument for pain management, anesthesia, and surgical care, improving patient outcomes and raising the quality of perioperative care.

Chapter 4

PHARMACOLOGY OF LOCAL ANESTHETICS

4.1 Types of Local Anesthetics

In the dynamic and ever-evolving area of anesthesiology, local anesthetics serve as a cornerstone, offering pain relief and enabling surgical operations with accuracy and effectiveness. This chapter goes closely into the numerous forms of local anesthetics, investigating their chemical properties, modes of action, therapeutic uses, and distinctive qualities. Understanding these substances is critical for enhancing anesthetic methods and maintaining patient safety.

Introduction to Local Anesthetics

Local anesthetics are a broad range of pharmacological drugs meant to elicit temporary loss of feeling in a particular location of the body without altering consciousness. They do this by inhibiting the conduction of nerve impulses in the targeted location. The efficacy of local anesthetics covers a broad variety of medical and dental treatments, from tiny skin lacerations to major surgical operations.

Chemical Classification of Local Anesthetics

Local anesthetics are roughly categorized into two primary types based on their chemical structure: amino esters and amino amides. This categorization not only impacts their pharmacokinetics and pharmacodynamics but also defines their therapeutic uses and propensity for allergic responses.

Amino Esters

Amino ester local anesthetics were among the first to be developed and utilized therapeutically. They are defined by the presence of an ester bond in their chemical structure. Common examples include:

Cocaine

- History and Use: Cocaine was the first local anesthetic identified and utilized in medical practice. Its powerful vasoconstrictive characteristics make it unique among local anesthetics.
- Mechanism of Action: Cocaine inhibits sodium channels, blocking depolarization and propagation of nerve impulses. Additionally, it decreases the reuptake of norepinephrine, adding to its vasoconstrictive actions.
- Clinical Applications: Primarily employed in ENT operations for its vasoconstrictive and anesthetic qualities, cocaine is currently less widely used owing to its propensity for misuse and systemic toxicity.

Procaine

- Development and Use: Developed as a safer alternative to cocaine, procaine (Novocaine) became extensively utilized in dentistry and minor surgical operations.
- Pharmacokinetics: Procaine has a quick onset and brief duration of action. It is processed by plasma cholinesterases, lowering the danger of systemic toxicity.
- Clinical Applications: Although less widely used nowadays, procaine is nevertheless applied in certain dental operations and as a spinal anesthetic.

Tetracaine

- Potency and Duration: Tetracaine is a very powerful ester local anesthetic with a longer duration of action compared to procaine.
- Clinical Applications: It is extensively used in spinal anesthesia and for topical anesthetic in ophthalmology and otolaryngology owing to its long-lasting effects.

Amino Amides

- Amino amide local anesthetics are characterized by an amide bond in their chemical structure, offering higher stability and longer duration of action compared to esters. Common examples include:

Lidocaine

1. adaptability: Lidocaine is one of the most extensively used local anesthetics owing to its quick onset, moderate duration of action, and adaptability.

- Mechanism of Action: Like other local anesthetics, lidocaine operates by blocking sodium channels and inhibiting nerve impulse transmission.
- Clinical Applications: Lidocaine is utilized in a number of contexts, including local infiltration, nerve blocks, epidural anesthesia, and as an antiarrhythmic drug.

Bupivacaine

1. Potency and Duration: Bupivacaine is noted for its great potency and lengthy duration of action, making it suited for treatments needing extensive anesthesia.
2. Clinical Applications: It is extensively used for epidural, spinal, and peripheral nerve blocks. Due to its cardiotoxic potential, care must be taken to prevent excessive systemic doses.

Ropivacaine

1. Safety Profile: Ropivacaine is identical to bupivacaine but with a lower risk of cardiotoxicity. It has a lengthy duration of action and is less prone to create motor blocks.
2. Clinical Applications: It is popular for epidural anesthesia during delivery and for postoperative pain control because of its safety profile.

Mepivacaine

1. Intermediate Duration: Mepivacaine has a somewhat longer duration of action than lidocaine but with comparable characteristics.
2. Clinical Applications: It is useful for peripheral nerve blocks and local infiltration, especially in individuals who may have contraindications to other amide anesthetics.

Mechanisms of Action

The principal method by which local anesthetics exert their effects is via the blockage of voltage-gated sodium channels. By binding to these channels, local anesthetics inhibit the entry of sodium ions, which is needed for the initiation and propagation of action potentials. This blocking leads to a reversible loss of feeling in the targeted location.

1. Binding Sites: Local anesthetics bind to the intracellular region of the sodium channel, especially at the S6 section of domain IV. This binding stabilizes the inactivated state of the channel, lengthening the refractory period and blocking nerve impulse transmission.
2. Use-Dependence: The effectiveness of local anesthetics is determined by the frequency of nerve impulses. High-frequency stimulation increases the chance of sodium channels being in an open or inactivated state, improving the binding and efficacy of local anesthetics. This trait is known as use-dependence or frequency-dependence.

3. Differential Sensitivity: Different nerve fibers demonstrate variable sensitivity to local anesthetics. Small, myelinated fibers (such as those responsible for pain and temperature sensitivity) are more vulnerable to blocking than bigger, unmyelinated fibers (such as motor neurons). This differential sensitivity allows for selective inhibition of sensory over motor function in specific therapeutic circumstances.

Pharmacokinetics of Local Anesthetics

The pharmacokinetic features of local anesthetics affect their onset, duration, and overall effectiveness. Key parameters impacting pharmacokinetics include lipid solubility, protein binding, pKa, and the rate of systemic absorption and metabolism.

1. Lipid Solubility: Highly lipid-soluble local anesthetics, such as bupivacaine and tetracaine, quickly permeate nerve cell membranes, resulting in a fast onset and powerful effects. However, they also have a larger risk for systemic toxicity.
2. Protein Binding: Local anesthetics having a high degree of protein binding, such as bupivacaine and ropivacaine, have a longer duration of action. Protein binding delays drug elimination and maintains effective drug concentrations at the site of action.
3. PKa and Ionization: The pKa of a local anesthetic affects its ionization at physiological pH. Local anesthetics with a pKa near to physiological pH have a greater fraction of the non-ionized form, permitting quicker penetration into nerve cells. Lidocaine, having a pKa of 7.7, has a quick onset owing to this feature.
4. Systemic Absorption and Metabolism: The place of injection considerably impacts the rate of systemic absorption. Highly vascularized regions, such as the intercostal space, result in fast absorption and increased plasma concentrations. Amino ester local anesthetics are metabolized by plasma cholinesterases, whereas amino amides undergo hepatic metabolism. The rate of metabolism and elimination

determines the duration of activity and potential for toxicity.

Clinical Applications and Considerations

The choice of local anesthetic and its administration rely on the individual clinical situation, intended duration of action, and patient characteristics. Here, we review several therapeutic uses and concerns for the use of local anesthetics.

Local Infiltration Anesthesia

1. Applications: Local infiltration anesthesia includes the injection of local anesthetic directly into the tissues around the surgical site. It is often used for minor surgical operations, dental treatments, and wound suturing.
2. Choice of Anesthetic: Lidocaine and mepivacaine are widely utilized because of their quick onset and moderate duration of action. For treatments needing extended anesthetic, bupivacaine may be employed.

Peripheral Nerve Blocks

1. Applications: Peripheral nerve blocks give localized anesthesia by administering local anesthetic near a particular nerve or nerve plexus. They are utilized for limb operations, pain management, and chronic pain disorders.
2. Choice of Anesthetic: The choice of anesthetic depends on the intended period of blockage. Lidocaine is good for short treatments, but bupivacaine and ropivacaine are preferable for lengthier procedures because of their sustained effects.

Epidural and Spinal Anesthesia

1. Applications: Epidural and spinal anesthesia entail the injection of local anesthetic into the epidural or subarachnoid area, respectively. These procedures are often utilized for delivery, lower abdominal, pelvic, and lower limb surgery.
2. Choice of Anesthetic: Bupivacaine and ropivacaine are often used for epidural and spinal anesthesia owing to their lengthy duration of action and differential sensory and motor blocking. Lidocaine is less typically used for spinal anesthesia owing to its shorter duration and possibility of transitory neurological effects.

Topical Anesthesia

1. Applications: Topical anesthesia includes the administration of local anesthetic to mucous membranes or skin. It is used for small treatments, such as suturing, diagnostic procedures, and alleviation of discomfort from minor burns or abrasions.
2. Choice of Anesthetic: Lidocaine and tetracaine are often used for topical anesthesia. Lidocaine patches and creams offer efficient pain treatment for localized skin problems.

Safety and Toxicity of Local Anesthetics

While local anesthetics are typically safe when administered carefully, they may induce systemic toxicity if absorbed in large doses or injected intravascularly. Understanding the indications, symptoms, and treatment of local anesthetic systemic toxicity (LAST) is critical for preserving patient safety.

1. Central Nervous System (CNS) poisoning: Early indications of CNS poisoning include circumoral numbness, tinnitus, and a metallic taste. As poisoning advances, patients may have convulsions, respiratory depression, and coma. CNS toxicity is addressed by delivering

benzodiazepines to reduce seizures and providing supportive care.
2. Cardiovascular Toxicity: Cardiovascular toxicity presents as hypotension, bradycardia, and arrhythmias. Bupivacaine is extremely cardiotoxic, with an increased risk of serious cardiac events. Management involves intravenous lipid emulsion therapy, which works as a lipid sink to absorb the local anesthetic and lower its plasma levels.
3. Allergic responses: Allergic responses to local anesthetics are uncommon but may occur, especially with amino ester anesthetics. Symptoms include redness, itching, bronchospasm, and anaphylaxis. Management entails stopping the anesthesia, delivering antihistamines, and providing supportive care.

Innovations and Future Directions

The area of local anesthesia continues to grow, with continuing research aimed at enhancing the effectiveness and safety of local anesthetics. Innovations include the discovery of novel drugs, medication delivery methods, and complementary therapy.

1. Long-Acting Local Anesthetics: Researchers are creating new long-acting local anesthetics that give sustained pain relief with minimal adverse effects. Liposomal versions of bupivacaine, for example, provide extended analgesia and lower systemic toxicity.
2. Adjuvant Therapies: Adjuncts like epinephrine, clonidine, and dexamethasone are utilized to increase the effects of local anesthetics. Epinephrine prolongs the duration of effect by limiting systemic absorption, whereas clonidine and dexamethasone improve analgesia and diminish inflammation.
3. Targeted Drug Delivery Systems: Advances in nanotechnology and drug delivery systems are opening the way for targeted and sustained release of local anesthetics. Nanoparticles, micelles, and hydrogels are being examined as carriers for local anesthetics, allowing precise delivery and controlled release.

Conclusion: Mastery in the Use of Local Anesthetics

The thorough knowledge of local anesthetics, from their chemical characteristics and mechanisms of action to their clinical uses and safety concerns, is crucial for any anesthesiologist or healthcare practitioner engaged in pain management and surgical treatment. Mastery in the use of local anesthetics not only promotes patient comfort and results but also enables the safe and successful delivery of anesthesia in varied clinical circumstances.

As the discipline continues to progress, remaining aware of the newest research, innovations, and best practices is vital for optimizing anesthetic administration and enhancing patient care. By utilizing the potential of local anesthetics, doctors may administer accurate, effective, and safe anesthesia, adding to the overall effectiveness of medical and surgical procedures.

4.2 Dosing and Administration

The prescription and administration of local anesthetics constitute a significant part of clinical practice, directly impacting the effectiveness, duration, and safety of anesthesia. Understanding the concepts underpinning dosage regimens and delivery strategies is critical for maximizing patient results and decreasing the risk of unwanted effects. This chapter presents a detailed investigation of the elements that affect the optimal dose and administration of local anesthetics, including pharmacokinetic considerations, patient-specific criteria, and practical procedures.

Principles of Dosing Local Anesthetics

Effective dosage of local anesthetics needs a compromise between obtaining enough anesthesia and avoiding toxicity. The dosage must be customized to the exact technique, patient characteristics, and the local anesthetic being utilized.

Pharmacokinetic Considerations

The pharmacokinetics of local anesthetics, including absorption, distribution, metabolism, and excretion, play a critical role in selecting the optimal dosage.

1. Absorption: The pace and degree of absorption of local anesthetics depend on the location of administration and the presence of vasoconstrictors. Highly vascular locations, such as the scalp or intercostal gaps, result in quick absorption and increased systemic levels, needing lower dosages to prevent toxicity. Conversely, weakly vascularized regions, including subcutaneous tissues, need greater dosages to establish adequate anesthesia.
2. Distribution: Once absorbed, local anesthetics are disseminated throughout the body. Factors affecting distribution include tissue binding, protein binding, and the lipid solubility of the anesthetic. Highly lipid-soluble anesthetics, such as bupivacaine, are more widely transported into tissues, increasing their duration of action.
3. Metabolism: Amino ester local anesthetics are quickly degraded by plasma cholinesterases, whereas amino amides undergo hepatic metabolism. The pace of metabolism impacts the duration of activity and the potential for systemic toxicity. Patients with hepatic impairment or abnormal plasma cholinesterase may need dosage changes to avoid buildup and toxicity.
4. Excretion: The principal route of excretion for local anesthetics is via the kidneys. Renal impairment may lengthen the elimination half-life, raising the risk of toxicity. Monitoring renal function is crucial in patients receiving repeated dosages or continuous infusions of local anesthetics.

Patient-Specific Factors

Individual patient factors considerably impact the dose of local anesthetics. These variables include age, weight, comorbidities, and concomitant medicines.

1. Age: Pediatric and geriatric individuals demonstrate distinct pharmacokinetic characteristics compared to adults. Children may need greater doses per kilogram of body weight owing to their bigger volume of distribution and quicker metabolism. Conversely, older people frequently need lesser dosages owing to diminished hepatic and renal function and higher susceptibility to local anesthetics.
2. Weight: Dosing local anesthetics depending on body weight is a standard practice, especially in young patients. However, in obese individuals, dosage based on target body weight rather than actual body weight may assist prevent overdose and toxicity.
3. Comorbidities: Conditions such as liver disease, renal dysfunction, cardiovascular disease, and neuromuscular disorders might influence the metabolism, excretion, and sensitivity to local anesthetics. Dose changes are recommended to limit the risk of adverse effects in these individuals.
4. Concurrent Medications: Drugs that modify hepatic enzyme activity or plasma protein binding may change the pharmacokinetics of local anesthetics. For example, drugs that activate cytochrome P450 enzymes may enhance the metabolism of amino amide anesthetics, requiring greater dosages to produce the intended effect. Conversely, medications that inhibit these enzymes may extend the effects and raise the risk of harm.

Techniques of Administration

The manner of administration has a vital influence in the effectiveness and safety of local anesthetics. This section covers numerous administration strategies, including local infiltration, peripheral nerve blocks, epidural and spinal anesthesia, and topical anesthetic.

Local Infiltration Anesthesia

Local infiltration includes injecting local anesthetic directly into the tissues surrounding the surgical site. This method is often used for minor surgical operations, dental treatments, and wound suturing.

- Procedure: The anesthetic solution is administered gently while withdrawing the needle to achieve uniform distribution. Aspiration before injection is required to prevent intravascular delivery. The amount and concentration of the anesthetic are regulated depending on the extent of the region to be anesthetized and the patient's characteristics.
- Advantages: Local infiltration is straightforward, needs minimum equipment, and delivers good anesthetic for superficial treatments.
- Challenges: The key problem is providing enough dispersion of the anesthesia to cover the whole operative region. Larger amounts may be necessary over large regions, raising the danger of systemic absorption and toxicity.

Peripheral Nerve Blocks

Peripheral nerve blocks require injecting local anesthetic near a particular nerve or nerve plexus to produce regional anesthesia. This procedure is utilized for operations involving the extremities, pain management, and chronic pain disorders.

1. Procedure: Using anatomical landmarks or ultrasound guidance, the needle is moved toward the target nerve. Aspiration is done to verify the needle is not in a blood vessel, followed by gradual injection of the anesthetic solution. Nerve stimulation or ultrasonography may confirm appropriate needle placement.
2. Advantages: Peripheral nerve blocks offer extended and focused analgesia, lowering the requirement for systemic analgesics and improving postoperative pain management.
3. Challenges: Accurate needle insertion is crucial to minimize nerve damage and guarantee good anesthetic. Ultrasound guiding has considerably improved the success rate and safety of peripheral nerve blocks.

Epidural Anesthesia

Epidural anesthesia includes injecting local anesthetic into the epidural area, providing anesthesia for operations affecting the lower belly, pelvis, and lower limbs. It is also extensively used for labor analgesia.

1. Procedure: The patient is positioned, and the skin is prepped with antiseptic solution. Using a loss-of-resistance approach, the epidural needle is moved into the epidural space. A catheter may be placed for continuous infusion or occasional bolus dosage.
2. Advantages: Epidural anesthesia gives great pain relief, the option to alter the dose of anesthesia, and low systemic adverse effects. Continuous epidural infusions enable sustained anesthesia and analgesia.
3. Challenges: Potential risks include unintentional dural puncture, resulting in a post-dural puncture headache, epidural hematoma, and infection. Proper technique and sterile measures are important to reduce dangers.

Spinal Anesthesia

Spinal anesthesia includes injecting local anesthetic into the subarachnoid area, enabling quick and substantial anesthesia for lower abdominal, pelvic, and lower limb procedures.

1. Procedure: The patient is positioned, and the skin is prepped with antiseptic solution. Using a spinal needle, the anesthetic is administered into the subarachnoid space after verifying cerebrospinal fluid (CSF) return.
2. Advantages: Spinal anesthesia offers quick onset and extensive sensory and motor blocking with a minimal amount of anesthetic. It is appropriate for short to moderate duration treatments.
3. Challenges: Potential risks include hypotension, bradycardia, post-dural puncture headache, and temporary neurological problems. Proper patient posture and diligent monitoring are necessary to

manage these hazards.

Topical Anesthesia

Topical anesthesia includes the administration of local anesthetic to mucous membranes or skin, giving surface anesthesia for simple operations.

1. Procedure: Local anesthetic creams, gels, patches, or sprays are administered to the target region. The length of administration and the concentration of the anesthetic dictate the depth and duration of anesthesia.
2. Advantages: Topical anesthetic is non-invasive and simple to give, making it excellent for small operations and pain management for localized skin disorders.
3. Challenges: The fundamental issue is getting enough penetration of the anesthetic to give effective anesthesia, especially for thicker skin or mucous membranes. Higher concentrations or longer application durations may be required.

Dose Calculation and Adjustment

Accurate dosage estimation and modification are required to provide the desired anesthetic effect while reducing the risk of harm. The following elements impact dosage calculation:

Maximum Recommended Doses

Each local anesthetic has a maximum suggested dosage to avoid toxicity. These dosages are depending on body weight and the particular anesthetic administered. For example:

1. Lidocaine: The highest suggested dosage without epinephrine is 4.5 mg/kg, while with epinephrine, it is 7 mg/kg.
2. Bupivacaine: The highest suggested dosage without epinephrine is 2.5

mg/kg, while with epinephrine, it is 3 mg/kg.
3. Ropivacaine: The highest suggested dosage without epinephrine is 3 mg/kg.

Volume and Concentration

The amount and concentration of the anesthetic solution dictate the degree and duration of anesthesia. Higher doses produce more powerful anesthesia but also raise the danger of systemic absorption and harm. The choice of volume and concentration should balance the necessity for effective anesthesia with the risk of unwanted effects.

Use of Vasoconstrictors

Adding vasoconstrictors, such as epinephrine, to local anesthetic solutions might increase the duration of effect and minimize systemic absorption. Vasoconstrictors do this by generating local vasoconstriction, limiting blood flow to the region and delaying the absorption of the anesthetic. However, care must be taken to prevent ischemia consequences, especially in end-artery locations like fingers, toes, and the penis.

Monitoring and Management of Toxicity

Despite cautious dose and administration, local anesthetic systemic toxicity (LAST) may develop. Early identification and timely care are critical for averting serious consequences.

Signs and Symptoms of Toxicity

The signs and symptoms of LAST may be categorized into central nervous system (CNS) and cardiovascular consequences.

1. CNS Effects: Early indications include circumoral numbness, metallic taste, tinnitus, and lightheadedness. As poisoning advances, patients may have visual abnormalities, muscular twitching, seizures, and loss of consciousness.

2. Cardiovascular Effects: Cardiovascular toxicity presents as hypotension, bradycardia, arrhythmias, and cardiac arrest. Bupivacaine, in particular, is linked with an increased risk of serious cardiac damage.

Management of Toxicity

The treatment of LAST comprises supportive care and specialized therapies to decrease systemic toxicity.

1. Airway Management: Ensuring a patent airway and delivering supplementary oxygen are crucial. In extreme situations, endotracheal intubation and mechanical ventilation may be essential.
2. Seizure Control: Benzodiazepines, such as midazolam or diazepam, are the first-line medication for controlling seizures. Propofol may be administered if benzodiazepines are unsuccessful.
3. Cardiovascular Support: Intravenous fluids, vasopressors, and inotropes may be required to control hypotension and bradycardia. In situations of cardiac arrest, advanced cardiac life support (ACLS) procedures should be followed.
4. Lipid Emulsion Therapy: Intravenous lipid emulsion therapy is a particular treatment for severe local anesthetic toxicity. Lipid emulsion works as a "lipid sink," absorbing the lipophilic local anesthetic and decreasing its plasma concentration. The normal dosage is an initial bolus of 1.5 mL/kg of 20% lipid emulsion, followed by an infusion of 0.25 mL/kg/min.

Case Studies and Clinical Scenarios

Case studies and clinical situations give useful insights into the actual implementation of dosage and administration concepts. The following examples show frequent scenarios seen in clinical practice.

Case Study 1: Local Infiltration for Minor Surgery

A 35-year-old guy arrives for excision of a tiny lipoma on his forearm. Local infiltration anesthesia is planned using lidocaine.

1. Patient Assessment: The patient has no relevant medical history and weighs 70 kg.
2. Dose Calculation: The highest recommended dose of lidocaine without epinephrine is 4.5 mg/kg, which is 315 mg for this patient. A 1% lidocaine solution has 10 mg/mL, hence the maximum volume is 31.5 mL.
3. Procedure: After prepping the skin with antiseptic, 20 mL of 1% lidocaine is injected progressively around the lipoma, maintaining equal distribution and aspirating before each injection to prevent intravascular delivery.
4. Outcome: The patient tolerates the surgery well with effective anesthesia and no evidence of toxicity.

Case Study 2: Peripheral Nerve Block for Upper Limb Surgery

A 60-year-old female needs carpal tunnel release surgery. A brachial plexus block is planned with ropivacaine.

1. Patient Assessment: The patient has a history of hypertension and diabetes and weighs 80 kg.
2. Dose Calculation: The highest recommended dose of ropivacaine without epinephrine is 3 mg/kg, which is 240 mg for this patient. A 0.5% ropivacaine solution has 5 mg/mL, hence the maximum volume is 48 mL.
3. Procedure: Using ultrasound guidance, 20 mL of 0.5% ropivacaine is injected around the brachial plexus. The patient is followed for evidence of effective block and systemic toxicity.
4. Outcome: The patient gets full anesthesia of the hand, with no side effects during or after the treatment.

Case Study 3: Epidural Anesthesia for Labor
A 28-year-old female in active labor seeks epidural analgesia.

1. Patient Assessment: The patient is healthy, with no contraindications for epidural anesthesia, and weighs 65 kg.
2. Dose Calculation: The maximum recommended dose of bupivacaine with epinephrine is 3 mg/kg, which is 195 mg for this patient. A 0.25% bupivacaine solution has 2.5 mg/mL, hence the maximum volume is 78 mL.
3. Procedure: After situating the patient and prepping the skin, an epidural catheter is placed using a loss-of-resistance approach. An initial bolus of 10 mL of 0.25% bupivacaine is delivered, followed by a continuous infusion of 0.1% bupivacaine with 2 mcg/mL of fentanyl at 10 mL/hr.
4. Outcome: The patient has adequate pain relief with little motor block, enabling her to engage in labor. No symptoms of toxicity are found.

Advancements in Dosing and Administration Techniques
Ongoing research and technological improvements continue to optimize the dose and delivery of local anesthetics. Innovations include real-time monitoring of anesthetic levels, innovative medication formulations, and enhanced delivery methods.

Real-Time Monitoring
Devices that enable real-time monitoring of local anesthetic concentrations in plasma and tissues are being developed. These devices may enable doctors to alter dose in real-time, maximizing anesthesia while avoiding toxicity.

Novel Drug Formulations
New formulations of local anesthetics, such as liposomal bupivacaine, enable sustained anesthesia with a single injection. These formulations release the anesthetic slowly, maintaining therapeutic levels over a long time and eliminating the need for recurrent dosage.

Advanced Delivery Systems

Nanotechnology and controlled-release devices are being researched to administer local anesthetics more accurately. Nanoparticles, micelles, and hydrogels may encapsulate local anesthetics, allowing targeted distribution and prolonged release, which may boost effectiveness and safety.

Conclusion: Mastery in Dosing and Administration

Mastery in the dose and administration of local anesthetics is vital for any anesthesiologist or healthcare practitioner engaged in pain management and surgical treatment. A detailed grasp of pharmacokinetic principles, patient-specific characteristics, and administration strategies is critical for ensuring effective and safe anesthesia.

By regularly upgrading their knowledge and abilities, doctors may optimize the use of local anesthetics, enhancing patient comfort and results. As the profession continues to evolve, adopting new technology and advances will further increase the accuracy and safety of local anesthetic delivery. The ultimate objective is to deliver high-quality anesthetic treatment, ensuring that patients enjoy the greatest possible experience throughout medical and surgical operations.

4.3 Adjuvant Medications

Adjuvant medicines have a vital role in increasing the effectiveness, duration, and safety of local anesthetics. By utilizing the pharmacological features of these adjuncts, doctors may customize anesthetic procedures to better meet the requirements of their patients, enhancing both procedural results and postoperative recovery. This chapter digs into the numerous adjuvant drugs used in combination with local anesthetics, studying their mechanisms of action, clinical uses, advantages, and possible hazards.

Introduction to Adjuvant Medications

Adjuvant drugs are substances that, when taken with main anesthetic agents, improve their effects. These adjuncts may be utilized to lengthen the duration of anesthesia, lower the needed dosage of local anesthetics, ameliorate adverse effects, and give extra analgesic advantages. The use of adjuvant drugs is a strategic strategy in anesthesiology, aiming to maximize patient care while avoiding possible consequences.

Common Adjuvant Medications

Several kinds of medicines are routinely used as adjuvants with local anesthetics. These include vasoconstrictors, opioids, alpha-2 adrenergic agonists, corticosteroids, and other medicines having specific modes of action.

Vasoconstrictors

Vasoconstrictors, such as epinephrine, are among the most often utilized adjuvants in local anesthetic.

1. Mechanism of Action: Vasoconstrictors function by constricting blood vessels at the site of injection, limiting blood flow and so delaying the absorption of the local anesthetic into the systemic circulation. This results in extended duration of action and a more concentrated impact at the site of administration.
2. Clinical Applications: Epinephrine is routinely administered to local anesthetics in operations requiring extended anesthesia, such as dental surgery, minor surgical procedures, and regional blocks. It is especially beneficial in locations with strong vascularity where quick absorption might lead to short duration and systemic toxicity.
3. Advantages: The principal advantages of vasoconstrictors are longer anesthetic, less systemic absorption, and decreased bleeding in the operative field. These actions increase the effectiveness and safety of local anesthetics.
4. Risks and Considerations: The use of vasoconstrictors might lead to possible consequences such as ischemia, especially in end-artery locations like the fingers, toes, and penis. Careful thought and

avoidance in these places are necessary. Additionally, people with cardiovascular issues may be at risk of systemic adverse effects such as tachycardia and hypertension.

Opioids

Opioids, such as fentanyl and morphine, are strong analgesics that may be utilized as adjuvants in regional anesthesia.

- Mechanism of Action: Opioids exert their analgesic effects by binding to opioid receptors in the central nervous system and peripheral tissues, regulating pain perception and transmission.
- Clinical Applications: Opioids are often given to epidural and spinal anesthetics to increase analgesia during and after surgical operations. They are also utilized in peripheral nerve blocks for enhanced pain management.
- Benefits: The addition of opioids to local anesthetics may give improved pain relief, lower the needed dosage of local anesthetics, and prolong the duration of analgesia. This may be especially effective in postoperative pain control.
- Risks and Considerations: Opioids involve a risk of side effects such as respiratory depression, nausea, vomiting, pruritus, and urine retention. The possibility for opioid-related side effects demands careful monitoring and dosage modification, particularly in individuals with reduced respiratory function or opioid sensitivity.

Alpha-2 Adrenergic Agonists

Alpha-2 adrenergic agonists, such as clonidine and dexmedetomidine, are efficient adjuvants that increase the effects of local anesthetics.

- Mechanism of Action: These drugs act on alpha-2 adrenergic receptors in the central and peripheral nervous systems, resulting in suppression

of norepinephrine release and associated analgesic and sedative effects.
- Clinical Applications: Alpha-2 adrenergic agonists are employed in many regional anesthetic procedures, including epidural, spinal, and peripheral nerve blocks, to extend anesthesia and enhance analgesia.
- Benefits: The use of alpha-2 agonists may greatly increase the duration of anesthesia, improve analgesia, and lower the needed dosage of local anesthetics. They also produce a sedative effect, which might be advantageous in some therapeutic circumstances.
- Risks and Considerations: Potential adverse effects of alpha-2 adrenergic agonists include hypotension, bradycardia, sedation, and dry mouth. These effects need careful monitoring and dosage adjustment, especially in individuals with cardiovascular instability.

Corticosteroids

Corticosteroids, such as dexamethasone, are increasingly being employed as adjuvants in regional anesthesia.

- Mechanism of Action: Corticosteroids exert their effects by regulating inflammatory responses and lowering the production of pro-inflammatory mediators. This leads to sustained analgesic effects and decreased postoperative pain and inflammation.
- Clinical Applications: Corticosteroids are used in peripheral nerve blocks, epidural injections, and intra-articular injections to extend the duration of analgesia and enhance postoperative pain management.
- Benefits: The use of corticosteroids may increase the duration of analgesia, minimize postoperative pain and inflammation, and enhance overall patient comfort and recovery.
- dangers and Considerations: Potential dangers of corticosteroids include immunosuppression, hyperglycemia, and delayed wound healing. These consequences demand careful attention and monitoring, especially in individuals with diabetes, infections, or reduced immunological function.

Other Adjuvants

Several different drugs are employed as adjuvants in local anesthetic, each with distinct processes and advantages.

1. Magnesium Sulfate: Magnesium sulfate serves as an NMDA receptor antagonist, giving extra analgesia and extending the effects of local anesthetics. It is used in epidural and peripheral nerve blocks to promote pain relief and minimize opioid usage.
2. Ketamine: Ketamine, an NMDA receptor antagonist, offers analgesic and anesthetic effects. Low-dose ketamine may be used as an adjuvant in regional anesthesia to increase analgesia and minimize opioid usage, especially in patients with chronic pain.
3. Sodium Bicarbonate: Sodium bicarbonate may be added to local anesthetics to raise their pH, resulting in speedier onset and enhanced quality of anesthesia. It is especially beneficial in procedures needing quick initiation of action.

Mechanisms of Action of Adjuvant Medications

Understanding the mechanisms of action of adjuvant drugs is vital for improving their usage in clinical practice. This section addresses the pharmacological interactions and routes by which these drugs increase the effects of local anesthetics.

Vasoconstrictors and Blood Flow Modulation

Vasoconstrictors such as epinephrine exert their effects largely by constricting blood arteries at the site of delivery. This vasoconstriction lowers blood flow, resulting to delayed absorption of the local anesthetic into the systemic circulation. The longer persistence of the anesthetic at the site of action results in increased duration and greater effectiveness. Additionally, vasoconstriction minimizes bleeding in the surgical field, giving a cleaner operating region and minimizing the likelihood of hematoma development.

Opioids and Pain Modulation

Opioids bind to opioid receptors in the central and peripheral nervous systems, regulating pain perception and transmission. By acting on these receptors, opioids limit the release of neurotransmitters involved in pain signaling, such as substance P and glutamate. This leads to lower pain perception and enhanced analgesia. When used as adjuvants, opioids increase the analgesic effects of local anesthetics, allowing for lower dosages and minimizing the risk of systemic toxicity.

Alpha-2 Adrenergic Agonists and Sympathetic Inhibition

Alpha-2 adrenergic agonists, such as clonidine and dexmedetomidine, work on presynaptic alpha-2 receptors to suppress the release of norepinephrine. This leads to reduced sympathetic output, resulting in analgesic and sedative effects. By boosting the effects of local anesthetics, alpha-2 agonists increase the duration of anesthesia and give further pain relief. Their sedative characteristics may also assist alleviate anxiety and increase patient comfort during treatments.

Corticosteroids and Inflammation Modulation

Corticosteroids exert their effects by regulating the inflammatory response and lowering the production of pro-inflammatory mediators such as prostaglandins and cytokines. This leads to reduced inflammation and discomfort, extending the analgesic effects of local anesthetics. Additionally, corticosteroids help minimize postoperative edema and enhance overall healing. Their usage as adjuvants in regional anesthesia gives long-lasting pain alleviation and better patient outcomes.

Clinical Applications and Techniques

The therapeutic uses of adjuvant drugs vary based on the kind of anesthetic and the unique demands of the patient. This section discusses the practical strategies and implications for employing adjuvants in various anesthetic treatments.

Epidural and Spinal Anesthesia

Adjuvant medicines are routinely used in epidural and spinal anesthesia to increase analgesia and lengthen the duration of anesthesia.

1. Epidural Anesthesia: In epidural anesthesia, adjuvants such as opioids, alpha-2 agonists, and corticosteroids may be added to the local anesthetic solution. This combination gives improved pain relief and increases the duration of anesthesia. Continuous epidural infusions may be customized with adjuvants to maintain good analgesia during surgery and the postpartum period.
2. Spinal Anesthesia: In spinal anesthesia, tiny amounts of adjuvants such as opioids and alpha-2 agonists may be added to the local anesthetic solution. This boosts the quality and duration of the block, providing excellent analgesia for lower abdomen and lower extremities procedures.

Peripheral Nerve Blocks

The use of adjuvants in peripheral nerve blocks may considerably increase the quality and duration of anesthesia and analgesia.

1. Single-Injection Blocks: For single-injection nerve blocks, adjuvants such as epinephrine, alpha-2 agonists, and corticosteroids may be added to the local anesthetic solution. This prolongs the duration of the block and gives longer pain relief.
2. Continuous Nerve Blocks: In continuous nerve blocks, adjuvants may be given to the local anesthetic infusion to maintain good analgesia. This is especially effective in postoperative pain treatment, as extended analgesia is essential to enhance recovery and limit narcotic intake.

Local Infiltration and Field Blocks

Adjuvants may also be utilized in local infiltration and field blocks to increase anesthesia for minor surgical operations.

1. Local Infiltration: Adding vasoconstrictors like epinephrine to the local anesthetic solution helps extend anesthesia and minimize bleeding in the operative region. This is beneficial in dental treatments, small skin surgery, and other surface procedures.
2. Field Blocks: In field blocks, adjuvants such as corticosteroids and alpha-2 agonists may be utilized to increase analgesia and lengthen the duration of anesthesia. This is especially beneficial in treatments needing lengthy pain management, such as hernia repairs and breast surgeries.

Benefits and Limitations of Adjuvant Medications

While adjuvant drugs provide significant advantages, they also come with restrictions and possible hazards. This section covers the benefits and problems related with their usage.

Benefits

1. Prolonged Anesthesia: Adjuvants may greatly lengthen the duration of local anesthetics, giving longer-lasting pain relief and lowering the need for repeated dosage.
2. Enhanced Analgesia: The inclusion of adjuvants may increase the quality of analgesia, enabling greater pain management during and after surgical operations.
3. Reduced Local Anesthetic Dose: By boosting the effects of local anesthetics, adjuvants allow for lower dosages, minimizing the risk of systemic toxicity and adverse effects.
4. Improved Patient Comfort: The use of adjuvants may improve patient comfort by providing effective pain relief and lowering anxiety and discomfort during treatments.

CHAPTER 4

Limitations and Risks

1. Side Effects: Adjuvants might induce side effects such as hypotension, bradycardia, respiratory depression, and nausea. These consequences need careful monitoring and control.
2. Complexity: The use of adjuvants adds complexity to anesthetic procedures, requiring a full knowledge of pharmacological interactions and associated consequences.
3. Patient Variability: Individual patient characteristics, such as medical history, comorbidities, and medication sensitivities, might impact the response of adjuvants, requiring tailored dose and monitoring.
4. Regulatory Considerations: Some adjuvants may have regulatory limits or recommendations that limit their usage in particular therapeutic circumstances.

Case Studies and Clinical Scenarios

Case studies and clinical situations give useful insights into the practical administration of adjuvant medicines in local anesthetic. The following examples show frequent scenarios seen in clinical practice.

Case Study 1: Epidural Anesthesia for Labor

A 30-year-old primigravida arrives in active labor and asks for epidural analgesia.

1. Patient Assessment: The patient is healthy with no contraindications for epidural anesthesia and weighs 70 kg.
2. Anesthetic Plan: An epidural catheter is inserted, and a solution of 0.1% bupivacaine with 2 mcg/mL fentanyl is produced. Dexmedetomidine is used as an adjuvant at a dose of 1 mcg/mL.
3. Procedure: After placement and skin preparation, the epidural catheter is placed using a loss-of-resistance approach. An initial bolus of 10 mL of the prepared solution is supplied, followed by a continuous infusion

at 10 mL/hr.
4. Outcome: The patient has adequate pain relief with little motor block, enabling her to engage in labor. No evidence of systemic toxicity or adverse effects are identified.

Case Study 2: Peripheral Nerve Block for Upper Limb Surgery

A 55-year-old guy needs surgical treatment of a distal radius fracture. A brachial plexus block is planned using ropivacaine with epinephrine and dexamethasone as adjuvants.

1. Patient Assessment: The patient has a history of hypertension and weighs 80 kg.
2. Anesthetic Plan: A solution of 0.5% ropivacaine with 1:200,000 epinephrine is prepared. Dexamethasone 4 mg is used as an adjuvant.
3. Procedure: Using ultrasound guidance, 20 mL of the prepared solution is injected around the brachial plexus. The patient is followed for evidence of effective block and systemic toxicity.
4. Outcome: The patient gets full anesthesia of the hand and forearm, with no side effects during or after the treatment. The block gives sustained pain relief, minimizing the requirement for postoperative narcotics.

Case Study 3: Local Infiltration for Minor Skin Surgery

A 45-year-old female arrives for removal of a basal cell carcinoma on the face. Local infiltration anesthesia is planned using lidocaine with epinephrine.

1. Patient Assessment: The patient has no relevant medical history and weighs 60 kg.
2. Anesthetic Plan: A solution of 1% lidocaine with 1:100,000 epinephrine is produced.

3. Procedure: After prepping the skin with antiseptic, 10 mL of the prepared solution is injected progressively around the lesion, maintaining equal distribution and aspirating before each injection to prevent intravascular delivery.
4. Outcome: The patient tolerates the surgery well with good anesthetic and minimum bleeding. No evidence of systemic toxicity is identified.

Advancements and Future Directions

Ongoing research and technical improvements continue to optimize the use of adjuvant medicines in local anesthetic. Innovations include innovative medicine formulations, real-time monitoring, and enhanced delivery methods.

Novel Drug Formulations

New formulations of adjuvants, such as sustained-release and liposomal preparations, offer longer and tailored benefits. These formulations may prolong the duration of analgesia and minimize the frequency of dose.

Real-Time Monitoring

Devices that enable real-time monitoring of medication concentrations in plasma and tissues are being developed. These devices may enable doctors to alter dose in real-time, maximizing anesthesia while reducing side effects and toxicity.

Advanced Delivery Systems

Nanotechnology and controlled-release technologies are being researched to distribute adjuvants more accurately. Nanoparticles, micelles, and hydrogels may encapsulate adjuvants, offering targeted distribution and prolonged release, which may boost effectiveness and safety.

Conclusion: The Strategic Use of Adjuvant Medications

The strategic use of adjuvant drugs is critical for enhancing the effectiveness, duration, and safety of local anesthetics. A detailed grasp of the pharmacological characteristics, mechanisms of action, and clinical uses of these adjuncts is critical for anesthesiologists and healthcare providers engaged in pain management and surgical care.

By regularly upgrading their knowledge and abilities, doctors may harness the full potential of adjuvant drugs, increasing patient outcomes and boosting the overall quality of anesthetic treatment. As the profession continues to evolve, adopting new technology and innovations will further enhance the use of adjuvants, ensuring that patients enjoy the best possible experience throughout medical and surgical operations. The ultimate objective is to deliver high-quality, tailored anesthetic treatment that matches the specific requirements of each patient.

Chapter 5

PREOPERATIVE ASSESSMENT AND PREPARATION

5.1. Patient Evaluation

Preoperative evaluation is a cornerstone of surgical treatment, laying the framework for safe and successful anesthetic management. Comprehensive patient assessment ensures that all relevant medical, surgical, and psychological aspects are examined, reducing risks and maximizing results. This chapter will go into the key components of patient assessment, preoperative testing, and informed consent, presenting a complete guidance for anesthesiologists and healthcare professionals.

History Taking

A comprehensive history is the first stage in patient assessment. It includes:

1. Medical History: Identifying chronic problems (e.g., diabetes, hypertension, cardiovascular disease), acute illnesses, and past surgical and anesthetic experiences. Special attention should be paid to any history of adverse responses to anesthesia or drugs.
2. Surgical History: Reviewing past operations and any difficulties that occurred, such as postoperative nausea and vomiting (PONV), difficult intubation, or protracted recovery.
3. Medication History: Documenting current medicines, including over-

the-counter pharmaceuticals, herbal supplements, and any known drug sensitivities. Understanding the patient's medication regimen is critical for predicting drug interactions and perioperative treatment.
4. Family History: Identifying any family history of anesthesia-related issues, such as malignant hyperthermia or pseudocholinesterase deficiency, which might guide the anesthetic approach.
5. Social History: Assessing lifestyle characteristics, including smoking, alcohol consumption, and recreational drug use, since they may affect anesthetic and surgical results.

Physical Examination

A focused physical examination is crucial to detect any concerns that might influence anesthesia and surgery. Key components include:

1. Airway Assessment: Evaluating the airway for predictors of difficult intubation, such as Mallampati score, neck movement, thyromental distance, and the existence of any anatomical anomalies.
2. Cardiovascular Examination: Assessing heart rate, rhythm, blood pressure, and symptoms of cardiovascular illness, such as murmurs, jugular venous distension, and peripheral edema.
3. Respiratory Examination: Evaluating respiratory rate, breath sounds, and symptoms of respiratory illness, such as wheezing, crackles, or diminished breath sounds.
4. Neurological Examination: Assessing mental state, motor and sensory function, and any indicators of neurological abnormalities that might influence anesthesia.
5. Other Systems: Performing a general examination to uncover any extra disorders that might impair the patient's perioperative course, such as abdominal distension, skin lesions, or musculoskeletal abnormalities.

Risk Stratification

Risk stratification is a vital step in preoperative evaluation, helping to identify individuals at elevated risk of perioperative problems. Several tools and grading systems are available, including:

1. American Society of Anesthesiologists (ASA) Physical Status Classification: A commonly used classification that categorizes patients based on their general health and the presence of systemic disorders.
2. Revised Cardiac Risk Index (RCRI): A method for estimating the risk of cardiac problems in non-cardiac surgery, based on criteria such as ischemic heart disease, heart failure, renal insufficiency, and diabetes.
3. STOP-Bang Questionnaire: A screening tool for obstructive sleep apnea (OSA), which may affect perioperative care and outcomes.

Functional Capacity

Evaluating the patient's functional capability is vital for measuring their ability to bear the physiological stress of surgery. This may be done through:

1. Activity Tolerance: Assessing the patient's capacity to undertake activities of daily life and participate in physical activity without developing symptoms such as chest discomfort, dyspnea, or weariness.
2. Metabolic Equivalents (METs): Using METs to assess functional capability. Patients able to execute activities involving more than 4 METs (e.g., ascending stairs, walking uphill) often have a decreased risk of perioperative problems.

Preoperative Optimization

Identifying and managing modifiable risk factors is an important component of preoperative preparation. This includes:

1. Medical Optimization: Managing chronic illnesses (e.g., lowering blood pressure, managing glucose levels in diabetics, stabilizing heart failure)

to lessen perioperative risks.
2. Medication Management: Adjusting medicines as required, such as maintaining beta-blockers and antihypertensives, monitoring anticoagulant treatment, and withholding pharmaceuticals that may increase bleeding risk.
3. Smoking Cessation: Encouraging patients to cease smoking at least several weeks before surgery to enhance respiratory and cardiovascular outcomes.
4. Nutritional Support: Assessing and optimizing nutritional status, especially in malnourished or fragile patients, to facilitate healing and recovery.

Patient Education and Expectations

Educating patients on the surgical and anesthetic procedures is vital for lowering fear and promoting compliance. This includes:

1. Preoperative advice: Providing explicit advice on fasting, medication management, and what to anticipate on the day of surgery.
2. Anesthesia strategy: Discussing the anesthetic strategy, including the kind of anesthesia (general, regional, or local), probable side effects, and postoperative pain management.
3. Healing and Rehabilitation: Informing patients on the anticipated healing period, possible problems, and the necessity of following postoperative instructions and attending follow-up visits.

Conclusion

A complete patient assessment is the cornerstone of safe and successful anesthetic treatment. By providing a complete history and physical examination, measuring functional ability, and addressing modifiable risk factors, anesthesiologists may reduce perioperative risks and enhance patient outcomes. Effective communication and patient education further increase the preoperative preparation, ensuring that patients are well-informed and prepared for their surgical experience.

5.2. Preoperative Testing

Preoperative testing is a crucial component of the preoperative examination, aiming at detecting any underlying problems that might affect anesthetic and surgical results. It comprises a mix of laboratory testing, imaging examinations, and specialist assessments suited to the specific patient's risk factors and the kind of surgery being done.

Guidelines and Best Practices

The selection of preoperative tests should be based on clinical standards and best practices, minimizing needless testing while ensuring that all important information is acquired. Several professional organizations, such as the American Society of Anesthesiologists (ASA) and the National Institute for Health and Care Excellence (NICE), make guidelines for preoperative testing.

Routine Laboratory Tests

Routine laboratory tests are routinely required for preoperative assessment, depending on the patient's age, medical history, and the kind of operation. These tests include:

1. Complete Blood Count (CBC): Evaluates hemoglobin, hematocrit, white blood cell count, and platelets. It is beneficial for diagnosing anemia, infection, and bleeding problems.
2. Basic Metabolic Panel (BMP): Includes electrolytes (sodium, potassium, chloride), glucose, blood urea nitrogen (BUN), and creatinine. It offers information on renal function, electrolyte balance, and metabolic condition.
3. Liver Function Tests (LFTs): Assess hepatic function and may identify liver disease, which may affect medication metabolism and coagulation.
4. Coagulation Profile: Includes prothrombin time (PT), activated partial

thromboplastin time (aPTT), and international normalized ratio (INR). It checks the coagulation state and may detect bleeding diseases.
5. Blood Glucose: Essential for diabetic patients and those at risk of hyperglycemia. It aids in controlling perioperative glucose levels.

Cardiovascular Testing

Cardiovascular testing is critical for individuals with known or suspected heart disease and those having high-risk operations. Tests include:

1. Electrocardiogram (ECG): A baseline ECG is indicated for patients with cardiovascular illness, those having major surgery, and older persons. It detects arrhythmias, ischemia, and other heart problems.
2. Echocardiogram: Indicated for individuals with symptoms of heart failure, valvular heart disease, or unexplained dyspnea. It examines heart function and structure.
3. Stress Testing: Used to assess myocardial ischemia and functional capability in individuals with substantial cardiac risk factors or symptoms indicative of coronary artery disease.
4. Cardiac Biomarkers: Troponins and B-type natriuretic peptide (BNP) may offer information on myocardial damage and heart failure, respectively.

Respiratory Testing

Respiratory testing is critical for individuals with chronic respiratory disorders, smokers, and those having thoracic or upper abdominal surgery. Tests include:

1. Pulmonary Function Tests (PFTs): Assess lung volumes, capabilities, and flow rates. They are helpful for assessing obstructive and restrictive lung disorders.
2. Arterial Blood Gas (ABG): Measures oxygenation, ventilation, and acid-

base status. It is intended for individuals with severe respiratory illness or those at risk of hypoxemia and respiratory failure.
3. Chest X-ray: Provides information on lung pathology, such as infections, tumors, and chronic lung disorders. It is not usually advised but may be effective in people with documented lung illness or severe risk factors.

Specialized Testing

Specialized testing may be necessary for particular patients and treatments, including:

1. Renal Function Tests: For patients with known or suspected kidney disease, tests such as creatinine clearance or glomerular filtration rate (GFR) offer extensive information on renal function.
2. Hematologic testing: For patients with known or suspected bleeding problems, testing such as platelet function assays, von Willebrand factor assays, and specific clotting factor levels are suggested.
3. Endocrine Tests: For individuals with endocrine diseases, such as thyroid function tests for those with thyroid illness, and cortisol levels for people with adrenal insufficiency.
4. Nutritional Assessment: For malnourished or high-risk individuals, tests such as serum albumin, prealbumin, and transferrin may offer information on nutritional status.

Risk-Based Testing Approach

A risk-based approach to preoperative testing guarantees that tests are ordered based on the patient's specific risk factors and the kind of operation being done. This method reduces superfluous testing and concentrates on acquiring therapeutically useful information.

1. Low-Risk Surgery: For low-risk operations (e.g., minor ambulatory

surgery), little testing is necessary for healthy individuals with no substantial comorbidities.
2. Intermediate-Risk Surgery: For intermediate-risk operations (e.g., major abdominal surgery), testing should be directed by the patient's medical history and clinical results.
3. High-Risk Surgery: For high-risk surgeries (e.g., heart surgery), thorough testing is typically essential to completely analyze and optimize the patient's health.

Preoperative Testing Algorithms

Utilizing preoperative testing algorithms helps shorten the assessment process and maintain uniformity in clinical practice. Algorithms often include patient parameters (age, comorbidities, functional status) and surgical factors (kind and length of operation) to inform testing choices.

Interpreting Test Results

Interpreting preoperative test findings needs a detailed awareness of normal values and the clinical relevance of anomalies. Abnormal results should be treated properly, including additional assessment, optimization of medical conditions, and contact with experts as required.

Patient-Centered Approach

A patient-centered approach to preoperative testing stresses tailored treatment and collaborative decision-making. It involves:

1. Patient Education: Explaining the purpose and possible effect of preoperative testing to patients, ensuring them understand the relevance of the assessment process.
2. Informed Decision-Making: Involving patients in choices concerning preoperative testing, including their preferences, concerns, and overall health objectives.
3. Minimizing worry: Reducing patient worry by giving clear informa-

tion, addressing concerns, and offering comfort regarding the testing procedure and its ramifications.

Conclusion

Preoperative testing is a critical component of the preoperative examination, giving important information to guide anesthetic and surgical planning. A thorough, risk-based strategy ensures that testing is customized to the individual patient, enhancing safety and results. By following clinical standards and best practices, and keeping a patient-centered focus, healthcare practitioners may successfully traverse the intricacies of preoperative testing and preparation.

5.3. Informed Consent

Informed consent is a crucial ethical and legal necessity in medical practice, especially in the setting of anesthesia and surgery. It guarantees that patients are adequately informed about their medical care, understand the risks and benefits, and have the ability to make autonomous choices on their treatment.

Principles of Informed Consent

The method of acquiring informed consent is based on three essential principles:

1. Autonomy: Respecting the patient's right to make informed choices regarding their healthcare.
2. Disclosure: Providing thorough and accurate information about the planned operation, including risks, benefits, alternatives, and possible results.
3. Comprehension: Ensuring that the patient understands the information offered, using clear and straightforward language, and addressing any questions or concerns.
4. Voluntariness: Ensuring that the patient's choice is made willingly,

without compulsion or undue influence.
5. Ability: Assessing the patient's ability to make informed choices, including criteria such as age, cognitive function, and mental health state.

Components of Informed Consent

Informed consent for anesthesia requires numerous critical components, including:

1. Nature of the Procedure: Explaining the kind of anesthetic (general, regional, local) and the processes involved in the administration procedure.
2. Risks and advantages: Discussing the possible risks and advantages of the planned anesthetic, including common and unusual problems, and the predicted results.
3. Alternatives: Presenting various anesthetic choices, including the risks and advantages of each, and explaining why a certain technique is advised.
4. Postoperative Care: Providing information on postoperative care and recovery, including pain management, probable side effects, and follow-up visits.
5. Questions and issues: Encouraging patients to ask questions and voice any issues they may have, and offering clear and thoughtful replies.

Process of Obtaining Informed Consent

The process of getting informed consent should be comprehensive and patient-centered, encompassing multiple steps:

1. First Discussion: Initiating the informed consent procedure at the preoperative exam, describing the planned anesthetic and answering any first queries.

2. Full description: Providing a full description of the anesthetic strategy, including the components listed above, and utilizing visual aids or textual materials as appropriate.
3. Assessment of knowledge: Assessing the patient's knowledge of the material delivered, asking them to repeat important points or describe their understanding in their own words.
4. Documentation: Documenting the informed consent conversation in the patient's medical record, including the information offered, the patient's questions and replies, and their choice for anesthesia.
5. Signed permission Form: Obtaining the patient's signature on a permission form that explains the important components of the informed consent conversation, ensuring that they understand and agree to the recommended anesthetic plan.

Special Considerations

Several particular issues may emerge in the context of informed consent for anesthesia, including:

1. Pediatric Patients: Obtaining informed permission from the parent or legal guardian, and including the child in the conversation as appropriate for their age and knowledge.
2. Older Patients: Assessing the competence of older patients to make informed choices, and including family members or legal representatives as required.
3. Emergency scenarios: In emergency scenarios when gaining informed consent is not practicable, recording the facts and the necessity for quick assistance is vital.
4. Language Barriers: Using interpreters or translated materials to guarantee that patients who speak a different language properly grasp the information offered.
5. Cultural Sensitivity: Being aware of and respecting cultural variations that may affect the informed consent process, and changing

the approach as required to enable successful communication and comprehension.

Legal and Ethical Considerations

Informed consent is not just an ethical imperative but also a legal need. Failure to get sufficient informed permission might result in legal implications, including allegations of medical malpractice. Key legal and ethical concerns include:

1. Legal Standards: Understanding the legal standards for informed consent in the relevant country, including the precise facts that must be revealed and the documentation requirements.
2. Patient Rights: Respecting patient rights and ensuring that the informed consent procedure is handled in a way that protects their rights.
3. Professional obligation: Recognizing the professional obligation of healthcare practitioners to seek informed consent and to guarantee that the patient's choice is recognized and honored.

Challenges and Solutions

Several problems may occur in the informed consent process, including:

1. Complicated Medical Information: Simplifying complicated medical information to ensure patient comprehension, utilizing analogies, visual aids, and simple language.
2. Anxiety and Stress: Addressing patient anxiety and stress, giving reassurance, and extending support throughout the consent process.
3. Time limits: Balancing the requirement for complete informed consent with time limits, prioritizing critical information and ensuring follow-up talks as required.
4. Disagreement and Refusal: Managing circumstances when the patient disagrees with the proposed anesthetic plan or denies permission,

considering alternate choices and respecting the patient's decision.

Case Studies and Clinical Scenarios

Case studies and clinical settings give useful insights into the practical implementation of informed consent in anesthesia. The following examples demonstrate frequent scenarios seen in clinical practice:

Case Study 1: Informed Consent for Elective Surgery

A 45-year-old female scheduled for elective laparoscopic cholecystectomy.

1. Initial Discussion: During the preoperative examination, the anesthesiologist outlines the intended general anesthetic, including the induction, maintenance, and recovery phases.
2. Detailed Explanation: The hazards of general anesthesia, including possible consequences such as aspiration, allergic responses, and postoperative nausea and vomiting, are described. Alternatives, such as regional anesthesia, are addressed.
3. Assessment of knowledge: The patient is asked to repeat essential statements and to express her knowledge of the anesthetic plan. Any misunderstandings are addressed.
4. Documentation: The informed consent talk is recorded in the medical record, and the patient signs the consent form, demonstrating her comprehension and assent.

Case Study 2: Informed Consent in Pediatric Anesthesia

A 6-year-old boy scheduled for tonsillectomy.

1. Initial Discussion: The anesthesiologist meets with the child's parents to explain the planned general anesthesia, answering their questions and concerns.
2. Detailed Explanation: The processes of the anesthetic process, includ-

ing induction with a mask, maintenance with inhalational drugs, and awakening from anesthesia, are detailed. Potential dangers, such as respiratory problems and emerging delirium, are mentioned.
3. Assessment of comprehension: The parents are asked to discuss their comprehension of the anesthetic plan, and any further questions are addressed. The youngster is also provided age-appropriate knowledge and reassurance.
4. Documentation: The informed consent conversation is documented, and the parents sign the permission form. The child's agreement is sought as suitable for his age.

Case Study 3: Informed Consent in an Emergency

A 65-year-old guy presenting with severe appendicitis necessitating emergent surgery.

1. Initial Discussion: The anesthesiologist briefly discusses the necessity for urgent general anesthesia with the patient and his family, emphasizing on the most relevant facts.
2. Detailed Explanation: Given the urgency, the discussion focuses on the immediate risks and advantages of general anesthesia. The necessity for timely response is highlighted.
3. Assessment of comprehension: The patient's comprehension is examined, and any pressing queries are answered. The family is participating in the discussion to give more assistance.
4. Documentation: The informed consent conversation is recorded, indicating the emergency nature of the circumstance and the necessity for accelerated consent. The patient signs the permission form if practicable, or verbal consent is recorded.

Future Directions and Innovations

Advancements in technology and developing ethical norms continue to impact the future of informed consent in anesthesia. Key areas of invention include:

1. Digital Platforms: Utilizing digital platforms for informed consent, including interactive modules, films, and electronic permission forms, can increase patient knowledge and speed the procedure.
2. Decision Aids: Developing decision aids, such as booklets, infographics, and mobile apps, to promote patient education and informed decision-making.
3. Shared Decision-Making: Promoting shared decision-making models that incorporate patients and their families in the anesthetic planning process, creating teamwork and trust.

Conclusion

Informed consent is a critical part of preoperative examination and preparation, ensuring that patients are fully informed and able to make autonomous choices regarding their treatment. By following ethical principles, legal requirements, and best practices, healthcare providers may successfully manage the intricacies of informed consent in anesthesia. Through clear communication, patient education, and a patient-centered approach, the informed consent procedure promotes patient trust, satisfaction, and results.

Chapter 6

TECHNIQUES OF LUMBAR EPIDURAL ANESTHESIA

6.1. Patient Positioning

The effective administration of lumbar epidural anesthesia rests on rigorous technique, and patient placement is a vital component of this procedure. Correct patient placement not only helps the identification of anatomical landmarks but also reduces patient pain and enhances the effectiveness and safety of the process. This chapter digs into the complete intricacies of patient posture, exploring numerous strategies, their benefits, and their consequences for clinical practice.

Importance of Patient Positioning in Lumbar Epidural Anesthesia

The fundamental purpose of patient placement in lumbar epidural anesthesia is to give optimum access to the epidural area while assuring patient comfort and safety. Proper orientation may considerably affect the ease of needle insertion, the precision of needle placement, and the overall success rate of the treatment. It also helps to decrease difficulties and promotes patient compliance, which is necessary for a smooth and effective anesthetic treatment.

Anatomical Considerations

Understanding the anatomical landmarks and their significance to patient placement is critical for practitioners practicing lumbar epidural anesthesia. The lumbar area of the spine has five vertebrae (L1 to L5), and the epidural space is inside the vertebral column, spanning from the foramen magnum to the sacral hiatus. Key anatomical markers are the iliac crests, spinous processes, and interspinous spaces. These landmarks aid the doctor in determining the optimum level for needle insertion, often between the L3 and L4 or L4 and L5 vertebrae.

Common Patient Positions for Lumbar Epidural Anesthesia

There are two basic postures utilized for lumbar epidural anesthesia: the sitting position and the lateral decubitus position. Each position has its own set of benefits and concerns, and the choice of position may rely on the patient's clinical state, the anesthesiologist's preference, and the particular needs of the surgical process.

Sitting Position

The sitting posture is commonly employed and has various benefits, notably in terms of ease of landmark recognition and needle insertion. In this posture, the patient is sitting with their feet supported on a stool or platform to provide stability.

Procedure:

- The patient sits on the edge of the bed or table with their feet on a stool.
- The back is arched forward to enhance the lumbar lordosis, providing a broader interspinous gap.
- The patient is encouraged to relax their shoulders and lay their arms on their thighs or a cushion put on their lap.
- The head is bent forward, and the chin is tucked towards the chest to further expand the interspinous gaps.

Advantages:

- Provides great visibility of anatomical markers, making it easy to locate the right intervertebral area.
- Facilitates patient participation, since they may be more readily led into the right posture.
- Allows for modifications to be performed rapidly if required, such as altering the degree of lumbar flexion.

Disadvantages:

- May be painful for certain individuals, especially those with back problems or restricted mobility.
- Requires patient participation and the capacity to hold the posture, which may be problematic for apprehensive or unwilling individuals.

Lateral Decubitus Position

The lateral decubitus position is another often utilized posture for lumbar epidural anesthesia. In this posture, the patient rests on their side with their knees pushed up towards their chest (fetal position).

Procedure:

- The patient lays on their side on the bed or table, with their hips and knees flexed.
- A cushion is put beneath the patient's head to ensure cervical alignment and comfort.
- The back is arched outward, and the shoulders are positioned perpendicular to the bed to optimize interspinous space opening.
- The patient's lower leg is flexed more than the upper leg to maintain the posture and avoid rolling.

Advantages:

- Often more comfortable for individuals, especially those with back problems or restricted movement.
- Can be useful in patients who are unable to sit straight, such as those with severe cardiovascular or pulmonary disorders.
- Reduces the risk of hypotension and vasovagal episodes that may develop in the sitting posture.

Disadvantages:

- Anatomical landmarks may be more difficult to palpate, especially in obese people.
- May be tough to acquire and maintain the right degree of lumbar flexion, especially in resistant or restless individuals.
- Limited access to the patient's airway in case of emergency, however this may be addressed with careful monitoring and preparedness.

Factors Influencing Position Choice

The choice of patient posture for lumbar epidural anesthesia may be impacted by various variables, including:

1. Patient Comfort: Patient comfort is vital. Patients with persistent back pain, arthritis, or other musculoskeletal problems may find certain postures more acceptable.
2. Anatomical Variability: Anatomical variances, such as body habitus and spinal abnormalities (e.g., scoliosis), might impact the ease of locating landmarks and placing the needle.
3. Clinical state: The patient's entire clinical state, particularly cardiovascular and respiratory health, might impact the choice of posture. For example, people with severe cardiovascular illness may be better suited

to the lateral decubitus posture.
4. Treatment kind: The kind and length of the surgical treatment may also affect posture choice. For extended treatments, preserving patient comfort and reducing movement is crucial.
5. Clinician Preference and Experience: The anesthesiologist's knowledge and comfort with a certain position might also play a factor in the decision-making process.

Enhancing Patient Positioning

Optimizing patient posture requires numerous ways to ensure the patient is both comfortable and adequately positioned for the treatment.

Communication and Patient Education

Effective communication with the patient is vital for attaining proper placement. Patients should be taught about the significance of the posture and what to anticipate throughout the surgery. Clear directions and reassurance may help minimize anxiety and promote participation.

Use of Positioning Aids

Positioning aids, such as cushions, folded towels, and positioning devices, may increase patient comfort and stability. For example, putting a cushion between the patient's legs in the lateral decubitus position may help preserve the fetal position and minimize lumbar lordosis.

Continuous Monitoring and Adjustment

Continuous monitoring and correction of the patient's posture throughout the surgery are vital. Small modifications to the degree of lumbar flexion or the position of the shoulders and hips may dramatically affect the ease of needle insertion and the success of the epidural block.

Case Studies and Clinical Scenarios

Case studies and clinical situations give useful insights into the practical application of patient placement for lumbar epidural anesthesia. The following examples demonstrate frequent scenarios seen in clinical practice:

Case Study 1: Epidural Anesthesia in an Obese Patient
A 45-year-old female with a BMI of 35 planned for elective hysterectomy.

1. Challenges: Difficulty in palpating anatomical landmarks owing to fat tissue, greater risk of positional discomfort.
2. Approach: The sitting posture was selected to assist landmark recognition. Positioning devices, such as a footstool and cushions, were utilized to support the patient's feet and arms, respectively. Continuous verbal advice and reassurance helped maintain the right stance.
3. Outcome: Successful diagnosis of the L3-L4 interspace, smooth needle insertion, and efficient epidural anesthesia with minimum pain for the patient.

Case Study 2: Epidural Anesthesia in a Patient with Severe Osteoarthritis
A 70-year-old guy with significant osteoarthritis of the spine planned for complete knee arthroplasty.

1. Challenges: Limited lumbar flexion, greater risk of discomfort and pain when placement.
2. Approach: The lateral decubitus posture was selected to optimize patient comfort. Extra padding and cushions were employed to support the patient's joints and preserve alignment. Gentle, progressive placement was attempted to decrease pain.
3. Outcome: Successful accomplishment of the fetal position, appropriate opening of the interspinous space, and efficient epidural block with minimum discomfort during positioning.

Case Study 3: Epidural Anesthesia in an Uncooperative Patient

A 35-year-old guy with a history of anxiety and panic episodes planned for inguinal hernia surgery.

1. Challenges: Difficulty in keeping posture owing to anxiousness and restlessness, greater chance of movement during needle insertion.
2. Approach: The seating posture was selected to provide for greater control and modifications. A gentle, soothing approach was employed to assist the patient into position. Distraction methods, such as engaging the patient in conversation and practicing relaxation exercises, were adopted.
3. Outcome: Successful alignment, agreeable patient, easy needle insertion, and successful epidural anesthesia with minimal anxiety-related problems.

Conclusion

Patient posture is a critical part of lumbar epidural anesthesia, directly affecting the effectiveness and safety of the surgery. By knowing the anatomical issues, determining the right position based on specific patient characteristics, and utilizing measures to maximize placement, doctors may optimize the results of lumbar epidural anesthesia. Effective communication, use of positioning aids, and continual monitoring are critical components of this procedure. Through careful attention to patient placement, healthcare personnel may assure a high level of care, promote patient comfort, and achieve good anesthetic results.

6.2. Needle Insertion Techniques

The accuracy and effectiveness of lumbar epidural anesthesia rely heavily on the expertise of needle insertion methods. This difficult treatment involves a detailed grasp of spinal anatomy, a precise technique, and a capacity to adjust to the patient's particular physiological features. This chapter presents a complete discussion of needle insertion procedures, concentrating on the concepts, procedural stages, and subtle tactics required for doctors to achieve effective epidural anesthesia.

Principles of Needle Insertion

The underlying premise of needle insertion in lumbar epidural anesthesia is to precisely implant the needle into the epidural area without piercing the dura mater. Achieving this involves a combination of anatomical understanding, tactile input, and procedural skill. The following concepts govern the technique:

1. Anatomical Understanding: Knowledge of the spinal column's anatomy, including the vertebrae, intervertebral discs, ligaments, and the epidural space, is vital. Familiarity with the common markers and their diversity among various patients helps accuracy.
2. Patient placement: As mentioned in Section 6.1, good patient placement is crucial. It promotes better identification of landmarks and offers a steady and accessible area for needle insertion.
3. Aseptic Technique: Maintaining proper aseptic technique during the treatment reduces infections. This involves good hand hygiene, use of sterile gloves, drapes, and sterilization of the puncture site.
4. Needle Selection: Choosing the suitable needle, often a Tuohy needle, is critical. The Tuohy needle's curved tip helps guide the epidural catheter and lowers the danger of dural puncture.
5. Tactile input: Recognizing the sensation of the needle traveling through distinct tissue layers offers vital input to minimize difficulties and ensure precise insertion.

Detailed Procedural Steps

1. Preparation

- Patient Education and Consent: Inform the patient about the operation, its risks, and advantages. Obtain informed consent, ensuring the patient

understands and agrees to continue.
- Positioning and Landmark Identification: Position the patient appropriately as mentioned in Section 6.1. Identify and label the anatomical landmarks, notably the iliac crests, spinous processes, and the interspinous gaps.
- Aseptic Preparation: Clean the puncture site with an antiseptic solution. Drape the area with sterile curtains, leaving the puncture site visible.
- Local anesthetic: Administer local anesthetic to the skin and subcutaneous tissues at the insertion site to lessen patient pain.

1. Needle Insertion Technique

- Initial Needle Insertion: Hold the Tuohy needle with the bevel pointing upward. Insert the needle at a 90-degree angle to the skin surface, aiming the interspinous area at the designated vertebral level (e.g., L3-L4 or L4-L5).
- Advancing Through the Ligamentum Flavum: Advance the needle gently and steadily. You will feel resistance as the needle travels through the interspinous ligament and subsequently the ligamentum flavum. The lack of resistance approach is widely employed here to confirm entrance into the epidural space.

1. Loss of Resistance Technique:

- Syringe Attachment: Attach a loss of resistance syringe filled with saline or air to the needle hub.
- Advancement: Advance the needle gently while giving mild pressure to the plunger. A quick lack of resistance suggests that the needle has penetrated the epidural area.
- Confirmation: Carefully check the absence of resistance by ensuring no cerebrospinal fluid (CSF) return, which would imply a dural puncture.
- Hanging Drop Technique: An alternate approach, the hanging drop technique, involves inserting a drop of saline at the needle hub. The

drop is pulled into the needle by negative pressure upon passage into the epidural space.

1. Finalizing Needle Placement

- Catheter Insertion: Once the needle is appropriately positioned, thread the epidural catheter through the needle into the epidural area. Advance the catheter to the required length, approximately 3-5 cm beyond the needle tip.
- Needle Removal: Carefully remove the needle while ensuring the catheter stays in place. Secure the catheter with adhesive tape to prevent displacement.
- Test Dose Administration: Administer a test dose of local anesthetic via the catheter to check accurate insertion and to rule out intravascular or intrathecal injection.

Advanced Techniques and Considerations

1. Ultrasound-Guided Epidural Anesthesia

Ultrasound guiding has emerged as a key technique in boosting the precision and safety of epidural needle placement. It gives real-time viewing of anatomical components, facilitating in the identification of the epidural space, particularly in patients with challenging anatomy.

Benefits:

- Enhanced Accuracy: Real-time imaging permits exact identification of the epidural space and lowers the risk of problems.
- Improved Safety: Minimizes the danger of dural puncture and unintentional intravascular injections.
- Better Patient Outcomes: Leads to increased success rates and improved

patient satisfaction.

Procedure:

- Preparation: Position the patient as for a standard epidural. Apply ultrasonic gel and position the transducer over the lumbar spine.
- Imaging: Obtain sagittal and transverse images to identify essential features, including the spinous processes, interspinous gaps, and the ligamentum flavum.
- Needle Insertion: Use the ultrasonography to guide needle insertion in real-time, verifying the needle's trajectory and penetration into the epidural space.

1. **Continuous Epidural Anesthesia**

Continuous epidural anesthesia includes the sustained delivery of anesthetic drugs via an indwelling catheter. This approach is excellent for long-duration procedures, postoperative pain control, and labor analgesia.

Advantages:

- Extended Pain Relief: Provides continuous pain relief, which may be modified depending on patient requirements.
- Flexibility: Allows for adjustment of anesthetic dosage and the inclusion of adjuvant drugs.
- Patient Comfort: Reduces the need for several needle insertions and promotes overall patient comfort.

Technique:

- Catheter Placement: Place the epidural catheter as indicated before.

Ensure it is properly taped to avoid dislodgement.
- Infusion System: Connect the catheter to an infusion pump or syringe driver to give a constant or intermittent bolus of anesthesia.
- Monitoring: Regularly check the patient for pain alleviation, sensory and motor block, and other adverse effects.

1. **Complications and Management**

Despite meticulous procedure, problems might develop during needle insertion for lumbar epidural anesthesia. Awareness and quick care of these consequences are crucial for patient safety.

Common Complications
Dural Puncture: Inadvertent puncture of the dura mater may lead to CSF leaking and post-dural puncture headache (PDPH).

1. Management: Conservative therapy includes bed rest, water, and painkillers. An epidural blood patch may be necessary for chronic PDPH.
2. Epidural Hematoma: Bleeding into the epidural space may induce compression of the spinal cord or nerve roots.
3. Management: Immediate assessment with MRI or CT scan. Surgical decompression may be indicated for severe instances.
4. Intravascular Injection: Accidental injection of anesthesia into a blood artery might induce systemic toxicity.
5. Management: Immediate termination of injection, supportive measures, and delivery of lipid emulsion treatment for local anesthetic systemic toxicity (LAST).
6. Nerve Injury: Direct damage to spinal nerves may result in acute or permanent neurological impairments.
7. Management: Monitor neurological function, offer supportive treatment, and refer to a neurologist if chronic impairments arise.

Case Studies and Clinical Scenarios

Case Study 1: Epidural Anesthesia in a Patient with Scoliosis

A 50-year-old female with scoliosis scheduled for spinal surgery.

1. Challenges: Anatomical malformation makes landmark recognition and needle placement problematic.
2. Approach: Use of ultrasound guidance to visualize the spinal architecture and guide needle placement.
3. Outcome: Successful needle insertion and epidural catheter placement with real-time ultrasound assistance, resulting in effective anesthetic and minimal problems.

Case Study 2: Epidural Anesthesia in a Pregnant Patient

A 30-year-old pregnant female in active labor demanding epidural analgesia.

1. Challenges: Anatomical changes related to pregnancy, include increased lumbar lordosis and edema of the epidural veins.
2. Approach: Careful placement in the lateral decubitus posture, use of a lower concentration test dosage to decrease the danger of intravascular injection.
3. Outcome: Successful pain alleviation with minimal maternal and fetal side effects.

Case Study 3: Managing Complications

A 45-year-old guy having lower limb surgery with epidural anesthesia exhibits indications of local anesthetic systemic toxicity (LAST).

1. Challenges: Immediate detection and treatment of systemic toxicity.
2. Approach: Cessation of anesthetic treatment, beginning of lipid emulsion therapy, and supportive measures include oxygen and intravenous

fluids.
3. Outcome: Rapid remission of symptoms and successful completion of the procedure using different anesthetic approaches.

Best Practices and Recommendations

1. Training and Skill Development

- Simulation Training: Utilize simulation-based training to strengthen needle insertion skills and management of problems.
- Continuing Education: Engage in continual professional development and attend workshops to remain informed with the newest methods and technology.

1. Patient-Centered Care

- Patient Communication: Maintain open and compassionate communication with patients, describing the process, resolving concerns, and offering reassurance
- Customized Approach: Tailor the procedure to the specific patient's anatomy, clinical condition, and preferences.

1. Quality Improvement

- Input and Evaluation: Regularly solicit input from patients and peers to discover areas for improvement.
- Clinical Audits: Conduct audits of epidural operations to monitor results, detect problems, and adopt remedial actions.

Conclusion
Needle insertion procedures for lumbar epidural anesthesia are a cor-

nerstone of good regional anesthesia treatment. Mastery of these methods demands a complete grasp of spine anatomy, rigorous procedural skills, and the capacity to adapt to particular patient features. By adhering to best practices, employing sophisticated technology such as ultrasound guidance, and emphasizing patient-centered care, doctors may achieve high success rates and reduce problems. Continuous learning, simulation training, and quality improvement activities further increase the competency and safety of epidural anesthetic techniques. Through attentive use of these ideas and practices, healthcare personnel may assure best results for patients having lumbar epidural anesthesia.

6.3. Catheter Placement and Securing

Catheter insertion and securing are critical procedures in the administration of lumbar epidural anesthesia, enabling continuous and regulated delivery of anesthetic drugs. This method involves accuracy, a detailed awareness of anatomical landmarks, and a precise approach to anchoring the catheter to minimize displacement or problems. In this chapter, we will go into the detailed intricacies of catheter insertion and securing, stressing the concepts, procedural procedures, and best practices essential for efficient lumbar epidural anesthesia.

Principles of Catheter Placement

The major purpose of catheter placement in lumbar epidural anesthesia is to ensure that the catheter is positioned precisely inside the epidural space, allowing for the efficient administration of anesthetic medications while limiting the risk of problems. The following concepts influence the catheter installation process:

1. Anatomical Accuracy: Understanding the exact location of the epidural space and associated anatomical structures is critical for correct catheter insertion.
2. Aseptic Technique: Maintaining rigorous aseptic conditions during

the process is crucial to avoid infections.
3. Patient Comfort and Safety: Ensuring patient comfort and reducing discomfort during catheter placement is a priority. The treatment should be completed with little pain and optimum safety.
4. Secure Fixation: Proper fastening of the catheter is crucial to avoid dislodgement and provide continuous and efficient analgesia.

Detailed Procedural Steps

1. Preparation

- Patient Education and Consent: Inform the patient about the catheter insertion process, its dangers, and advantages. Obtain informed consent, ensuring the patient understands and agrees to the operation.
- Patient Positioning: Position the patient appropriately, as specified in Section 6.1. Proper positioning promotes simpler identification of landmarks and offers a solid field for catheter implantation.
- Aseptic Preparation: Clean the puncture site with an antiseptic solution. Use sterile gloves, drapes, and other appropriate sterile equipment to maintain aseptic conditions.

C
atheter Placement Technique

1. Needle Insertion: Follow the needle insertion procedure as outlined in Section 6.2. Once the epidural space is discovered using the loss of resistance method or the hanging drop technique, the needle should be properly positioned.

Catheter Insertion:

1. **Catheter Preparation:** Prepare the epidural catheter, ensuring it is clear of air bubbles and adequately primed with sterile saline.
2. **Threading the Catheter:** Gently thread the catheter through the Tuohy needle into the epidural area. The catheter should be pushed 3-5 cm beyond the needle tip to ensure it is well into the epidural space.
3. **Resistance Check:** Ensure that there is minimum resistance when threading the catheter. If resistance is experienced, remove the catheter slightly and try to re-thread. Avoid pushing the catheter, since this may cause kinking or injury.

Needle Removal:

1. **Stabilizing the Catheter:** Once the catheter is in place, hold it tightly to avoid dislodgement.
2. **Needle Withdrawal:** Carefully remove the Tuohy needle while maintaining the catheter in place. Ensure the catheter stays stable and does not shift during needle extraction.

Securing the Catheter

Proper securing of the epidural catheter is crucial to preserve its position and assure continuous analgesia. The following stages explain the method of securing the catheter:

1. **Catheter location Confirmation:** Before attaching the catheter, assess its location by aspirating gently to look for blood or cerebrospinal fluid (CSF). The lack of blood or CSF confirms proper placement.

Dressing and Taping:

1. **Sterile Dressing:** Apply a sterile dressing to the catheter insertion site.

Ensure the dressing is secure and covers the puncture site entirely
2. Taping the Catheter: Use adhesive tape to fix the catheter. The tape should be placed in a way that eliminates kinking and allows for some flexibility. Ensure the catheter is secured tightly to the patient's skin without creating pain.

Additional Securing Methods:

1. Tunneling: In certain circumstances, tunneling the catheter subcutaneously for a short distance before it leaves the skin might give extra security and lessen the chance of unintentional dislodgement.
2. Adhesive Anchors: Use adhesive anchors or securement devices developed for epidural catheters to give extra support.
3. Labeling: Clearly mark the catheter with information such as the insertion date, catheter length, and any other pertinent facts. This aids in monitoring and managing the catheter throughout its usage.

Continuous Infusion and Monitoring

Once the catheter is secured, continuous or intermittent infusion of anesthetic drugs may be delivered. The following factors are required for successful and safe infusion:

1. Infusion System Setup: Connect the epidural catheter to an infusion pump or syringe driver. Ensure the infusion device is correctly calibrated and configured according to the authorized dose plan.
2. Initial Test Dose: Administer an initial test dose of local anesthetic to establish the catheter's insertion and rule out intravascular or intrathecal injection. Monitor the patient for any adverse reactions or problems.
3. Continuous Monitoring: Regularly check the patient's pain levels, sensory and motor block, and vital signs. Adjust the infusion rate

and anesthetic dosage as required to maintain good analgesia.
4. Complication Management: Be watchful for possible complications such as catheter migration, infection, or local anesthetic systemic toxicity (LAST). Promptly resolve any concerns that occur to protect patient safety.

Case Studies and Clinical Scenarios

Case Study 1: Epidural Catheter Placement in a Patient with Obesity

A 55-year-old guy with a body mass index (BMI) of 40, scheduled for lower extremities surgery.

1. Challenges: Increased adipose tissue making landmark recognition and catheter insertion harder.
2. Approach: Use of ultrasound guidance to visualize anatomical features and guide needle and catheter placement.
3. Outcome: Successful catheter insertion with ultrasound guidance, resulting in effective anesthetic and few problems.

Case Study 2: Epidural Catheter Placement for Labor Analgesia

A 30-year-old pregnant female in active labor demanding epidural analgesia.

1. Challenges: Anatomical changes related to pregnancy, including increased lumbar lordosis and epidural vein engorgement.
2. Approach: Careful placement in the lateral decubitus posture, use of a lower concentration test dosage to decrease the danger of intravascular injection.
3. Outcome: Effective pain treatment with minimal maternal and fetal side effects, resulting in a good labor experience.

Case Study 3: Managing Epidural Catheter Dislodgement

A 45-year-old female having thoracic surgery with epidural anesthesia reports poor pain alleviation postoperatively.

1. Challenges: Suspected catheter dislodgement producing insufficient analgesia.

- Approach: Assessment of catheter placement utilizing imaging (X-ray or fluoroscopy) to confirm dislodgement. Re-insertion of the catheter under guided imaging.
- Outcome: Restored effective analgesia after re-positioning the catheter, resulting in better pain control and patient comfort.

Advanced Techniques and Innovations

Use of Epidural Catheter Securement Devices

Innovations in catheter securement devices have enhanced the stability and dependability of epidural catheters. These devices offer better fixation, lowering the likelihood of catheter movement and related problems.

1. Adhesive Securement Devices: These devices have adhesive pads and locking mechanisms that firmly bind the catheter to the skin. They provide flexibility, lowering the chance of kinking or dislodgement.
2. Subcutaneous Anchors: Subcutaneous anchoring devices are meant to attach the catheter under the skin, giving greater stability and lowering the danger of external dislodgement.
3. Integrated Infusion Systems: Advanced infusion systems with integrated catheter securement features provide a simplified approach to epidural anesthesia, combining secure fixation with accurate medication administration.

Patient-Centered Care and Communication

Effective communication and patient-centered treatment are important in ensuring the success of epidural catheter insertion and securing. Engaging with patients, addressing their worries, and offering comprehensive explanations of the treatment contribute to a happy experience and excellent results.

1. Patient Education: Educate patients about the catheter placement process, possible hazards, and what to anticipate during and after the treatment. Provide textual material and answer any queries they may have.
2. Empathy and Reassurance: Approach the procedure with empathy, noting the patient's concern and giving reassurance throughout the process.
3. Post-Procedure Instructions: Give explicit post-procedure instructions on activity limits, indicators of problems, and when to seek medical assistance

Quality Improvement and Best Practices

- Training and Skill Development
- Simulation Training: Utilize simulation-based training to strengthen catheter placement abilities and improve the management of problems.
- Continuing Education: Engage in continual professional development and attend seminars to remain informed with the newest methods and technology.

Standardization and Protocols

- Standardized procedures: Develop and execute standardized procedures for epidural catheter insertion and securing to promote consistency and safety across clinical settings.

- Clinical Audits: Conduct frequent audits of epidural operations to assess results, identify areas for improvement, and implement remedial actions.

Feedback and Evaluation

- Patient input: Regularly solicit input from patients on their experience with epidural catheter placement and analgesia. Use this input to develop approaches and improve patient care.
- Peer Review: Engage in peer review and collaborative practice to exchange information, debate problematic situations, and strengthen clinical abilities.

Conclusion

Catheter insertion and securing are key components of effective lumbar epidural anesthesia, requiring a cautious approach and a complete awareness of anatomical, procedural, and patient-centered factors. By following best practices, employing innovative technology, and emphasizing patient comfort and safety, doctors may achieve high success rates and excellent results in epidural anesthesia. Continuous learning, quality improvement activities, and good communication further increase the competency and dependability of epidural catheter insertion and securing. Through attentive use of these concepts and procedures, healthcare personnel may assure the safe and successful administration of epidural anesthesia, leading to enhanced patient experiences and clinical results.

Chapter 7

EQUIPMENT AND MATERIALS

7.1. Needles and Catheters

The delivery of lumbar epidural anesthesia rests on the right selection and usage of specific equipment and materials. Among the most crucial of them are the needles and catheters, which play key roles in assuring successful administration of anesthetic drugs to the epidural area. This chapter digs into the extensive details of the many kinds of needles and catheters used in lumbar epidural anesthesia, exploring their design, functioning, and the principles governing their usage. By knowing the properties and uses of these critical instruments, doctors may increase the accuracy, safety, and effectiveness of epidural anesthetic.

Anatomy and Functionality of Needles in Epidural Anesthesia

The selection of needles for lumbar epidural anesthesia is a vital stage that determines the effectiveness of the treatment. The following sections address the design, kinds, and utilization of needles in epidural anesthesia.

Design Features of Epidural Needles

1. Bevel Type: Epidural needles are often constructed with a curved or blunt bevel, which assists in lowering the danger of dural puncture and

permits simpler insertion into the epidural area.
2. Tuohy Needle: The most often used needle for epidural anesthesia, with a curved, blunt tip that leads the catheter into the spinal region.
3. Hustead Needle: Similar to the Tuohy needle but with a less noticeable curvature, allowing an option depending on clinical choice.
4. Crawford Needle: Features a straight, thin-walled shape with a small bevel, offering another alternative for particular clinical settings.
5. Gauge and Length: Epidural needles exist in various gauges and lengths to fit varied patient anatomies and procedural needs.
6. Gauge: Commonly used gauges range from 16 to 18. Larger gauges (e.g., 16G) permit simpler catheter insertion, whereas smaller gauges (e.g., 18G) may be chosen for individuals with smaller anatomical features.
7. Length: Needle lengths generally vary from 8 to 18 cm, with longer needles utilized for individuals with more adipose tissue or deeper epidural spaces.
8. Stylet: A stylet is used to occlude the lumen of the needle during insertion, preventing tissue or blood from clogging the needle. The stylet is withdrawn after the epidural space is reached.

Types of Epidural Needles

1. Tuohy Needle: The Tuohy needle, with its curved tip, is meant to route the catheter into the epidural area, limiting the danger of dural puncture. It is the most extensively used needle for lumbar epidural anesthesia.
2. Hustead Needle: Similar to the Tuohy needle, the Hustead needle has a less prominent curvature, giving a somewhat different insertion approach while still delivering good catheter guiding.
3. Crawford Needle: The Crawford needle boasts a straight shape with a small bevel, allowing a new approach for physicians who prefer a less curved insertion method.
4. Weiss Needle: The Weiss needle, with its distinctive design, is employed in various therapeutic settings when a more specialist approach is

necessary. It gives an option for tough anatomical circumstances.

Principles of Needle Insertion

The effective insertion of an epidural needle demands a detailed awareness of the anatomical landmarks and meticulous technique. The following concepts govern needle insertion:

1. Identification of Landmarks: Accurate identification of anatomical landmarks, such as the iliac crests, spinous processes, and interspinous spaces, is crucial for exact needle placement.
2. Aseptic Technique: Maintaining rigorous aseptic conditions during the process is crucial to avoid infections.
3. Patient placement: Proper patient placement, such as the lateral decubitus or sitting posture, promotes simpler identification of landmarks and offers a stable field for needle insertion.
4. Needle Insertion Technique: The needle is placed at a 90-degree angle to the skin, with the bevel pointing cephalad. The needle is advanced gently and cautiously, utilizing the loss of resistance method or the hanging drop technique to detect the epidural space.

Catheters in Epidural Anesthesia

Epidural catheters serve a critical function in providing continuous or intermittent doses of anesthetic drugs into the epidural area. The following sections address the design, kinds, and use of epidural catheters.

Design Features of Epidural Catheters

1. Material: Epidural catheters are often fashioned from flexible, biocompatible materials such as polyurethane or nylon. These materials offer a blend of flexibility and strength, enabling the catheter to cross the epidural area without kinking.
2. Lumens: Catheters may have single or several lumens, with multi-lumen catheters allowing for the administration of various agents

concurrently.
3. Tip Design: The tip of the catheter may be open-ended or closed-ended with several side holes. Open-ended catheters give a direct conduit for the anesthetic chemical, whereas closed-ended catheters with side perforations allow a more dispersed administration.

Types of Epidural Catheters

1. Single-Lumen Catheters: Single-lumen catheters are the most often used form, offering an easy and effective technique for administering anesthetic drugs into the epidural area.
2. Multi-Lumen Catheters: Multi-lumen catheters, having two or more lumens, allow for the simultaneous administration of multiple drugs, such as local anesthetics and opioids, offering superior pain control.
3. Wire-Reinforced Catheters: These catheters contain a wire reinforcement that boosts their strength and lowers the chance of kinking, making them suited for patients with complex anatomical features.
4. Catheters with Closed Tip and Side Holes: These catheters feature a closed tip with many side holes, giving a more diffuse distribution of the anesthetic drug and lowering the danger of catheter migration.

Principles of Catheter Insertion
The effective placement of an epidural catheter demands precise skill and attention to detail. The following principles govern catheter insertion:

1. Needle Insertion: Follow the needle insertion procedure as mentioned before. Once the epidural space is recognized, the needle should be properly positioned.

Catheter Insertion:

- Preparation: Prepare the catheter, ensuring it is clear of air bubbles and adequately primed with sterile saline.
- Threading the Catheter: Gently thread the catheter through the needle into the epidural area. The catheter should be pushed 3-5 cm beyond the needle tip to ensure it is well into the epidural space.
- Resistance Check: Ensure little resistance when threading the catheter. If resistance is experienced, remove the catheter slightly and try to re-thread. Avoid straining the catheter to avoid kinking or injury.

Needle Removal:

1. Stabilizing the Catheter: Once the catheter is in place, hold it tightly to avoid dislodgement.
2. Needle Withdrawal: Carefully extract the needle while maintaining the catheter in place. Ensure the catheter stays stable and does not shift during needle extraction.

Securing the Epidural Catheter

Proper securing of the epidural catheter is crucial to preserve its position and assure continuous analgesia. The following stages explain the method of securing the catheter:

1. Catheter location Confirmation: Before attaching the catheter, assess its location by aspirating gently to look for blood or cerebrospinal fluid (CSF). The lack of blood or CSF confirms proper placement.

Dressing and Taping:

1. Sterile Dressing: Apply a sterile dressing to the catheter insertion site. Ensure the dressing is secure and covers the puncture site entirely.
2. Taping the Catheter: Use adhesive tape to fix the catheter. The tape should be placed in a way that eliminates kinking and allows for some

flexibility. Ensure the catheter is secured tightly to the patient's skin without creating pain.

Additional Securing Methods:

1. Tunneling: In certain circumstances, tunneling the catheter subcutaneously for a short distance before it leaves the skin might give extra security and lessen the chance of unintentional dislodgement.
2. Adhesive Anchors: Use adhesive anchors or securement devices developed for epidural catheters to give extra support.
3. Labeling: Clearly mark the catheter with information such as the insertion date, catheter length, and any other pertinent facts. This aids in monitoring and managing the catheter throughout its usage.

Continuous Infusion and Monitoring

Once the catheter is secured, continuous or intermittent infusion of anesthetic drugs may be delivered. The following factors are required for successful and safe infusion:

1. Infusion System Setup: Connect the epidural catheter to an infusion pump or syringe driver. Ensure the infusion device is correctly calibrated and configured according to the authorized dose plan.
2. Initial Test Dose: Administer an initial test dose of local anesthetic to establish the catheter's insertion and rule out intravascular or intrathecal injection. Monitor the patient for any adverse reactions or problems.
3. Continuous Monitoring: Regularly check the patient's pain levels, sensory and motor block, and vital signs. Adjust the infusion rate and anesthetic dosage as required to maintain good analgesia.
4. Complication Management: Be watchful for possible complications such as catheter migration, infection, or local anesthetic systemic toxicity (LAST). Promptly resolve any concerns that occur to protect patient safety.

Case Studies and Clinical Scenarios

Case Study 1: Epidural Catheter Placement in a Patient with Obesity

A 55-year-old guy with a body mass index (BMI) of 40 arrived for elective lumbar spine surgery. The patient had a history of severe back pain and hypertension. Given his weight, the anesthesiologist expected difficulty in recognizing anatomical landmarks and putting the epidural catheter.

Approach and Outcome:

1. Needle Selection: A 16G Tuohy needle was used for its larger gauge and simplicity of catheter insertion.
2. Patient Positioning: The patient was positioned in the sitting posture with the help of an assistant to maximize landmark recognition.
3. Landmark Identification: Palpation of the iliac crests and spinous processes was problematic owing to adipose tissue. Ultrasound guidance was utilized to examine the interspinous space and confirm the appropriate insertion placement.
4. Catheter Insertion: The needle was inserted utilizing the loss of resistance approach. Once the epidural space was found, a wire-reinforced catheter was inserted easily without difficulty.
5. Securing the Catheter: The catheter was fixed using adhesive anchors and an extra tunneling approach to limit the danger of dislodgement.
6. Monitoring and Infusion: Continuous infusion of bupivacaine was provided, giving excellent analgesia throughout the surgical operation.

The combination of ultrasound guidance and a wire-reinforced catheter enabled safe insertion and securement of the epidural catheter, resulting in excellent pain control for the patient.

Case Study 2: Epidural Analgesia in Labor and Delivery

A 30-year-old primigravida at 39 weeks of gestation appeared in active labor. She wanted epidural anesthesia for pain alleviation. The patient had no substantial medical history and was in excellent health.

Approach and Outcome:

1. Needle Selection: An 18G Tuohy needle was selected for its balance of size and simplicity of catheter insertion.
2. Patient Positioning: The patient was positioned in the lateral decubitus position with her back arched to enlarge the interspinous gaps.
3. Landmark Identification: Palpation of the iliac crests and lumbar vertebrae was done to locate the insertion point at the L3-L4 interspace.
4. Catheter Insertion: The needle was advanced utilizing the loss of resistance approach. A single-lumen catheter was threaded 5 cm beyond the needle tip with little difficulty.
5. Securing the Catheter: The catheter was fixed using sterile dressing and adhesive tape, providing stability without causing pain to the patient.
6. Monitoring and Infusion: An initial test dosage of lidocaine was delivered, followed by continuous infusion of a mixture of bupivacaine and fentanyl. The patient got great pain relief and was able to relax comfortably throughout birth.

The prompt and efficient implantation of the epidural catheter provided excellent analgesia, increasing the patient's labor and delivery experience.

Advances in Epidural Needle and Catheter Technology

Recent developments in epidural needle and catheter technologies have significantly enhanced the safety and effectiveness of lumbar epidural anesthesia. The following inventions are noteworthy:

1. Echogenic Needles: Echogenic needles are engineered with surfaces that reflect ultrasound waves, boosting their visibility under ultrasound guidance. This technique allows accurate needle insertion, particularly in patients with complex anatomical features.
2. Integrated Catheter Systems: New catheter systems include sensors and feedback mechanisms to offer real-time data on catheter placement and operation. These devices increase accuracy and minimize the danger of problems.
3. Flexible Catheters with Improved Biocompatibility: Advances in mate-

rials science have led to the creation of more flexible and biocompatible catheters, minimizing the risk of tissue irritation and enhancing patient comfort.

Conclusion

The full knowledge of needles and catheters in lumbar epidural anesthesia is crucial for the efficient administration of this analgesic treatment. By choosing the proper needles and catheters, following precise insertion procedures, and leveraging new technology, doctors may optimize the safety, effectiveness, and patient experience of epidural anesthesia. Continuous education, clinical practice, and innovation in equipment design will further develop the discipline, assuring best results for patients having lumbar epidural anesthesia. Through attentive application of these concepts and approaches, healthcare personnel may give high-quality treatment and effective pain management in a range of clinical settings.

7.2. Epidural Kits

The administration of lumbar epidural anesthesia is a sophisticated and precise technique that demands a full grasp of the equipment and materials involved. Central to this procedure are epidural kits, which are precisely engineered to include all the required components for providing epidural anesthesia. This chapter gives a comprehensive study of the many parts contained in epidural kits, the reasoning for their inclusion, and the principles guiding their usage. By knowing the contents and uses of epidural kits, doctors may increase the safety, efficiency, and efficacy of epidural anesthetic treatments.

Overview of Epidural Kits

Epidural kits are standardized packages that comprise all the key instruments and supplies needed for the safe and successful delivery of epidural anesthesia. These kits are intended to expedite the preparation and execution of the surgery, ensuring that professionals have instant access to everything they need. The components of epidural kits often contain needles, catheters, syringes, filters, local anesthetics, antiseptic solutions, drapes, and other auxiliary materials.

Standard Components of Epidural Kits

1. Epidural Needle: The needle is a vital component for reaching the epidural region. Common varieties included in epidural kits include Tuohy, Hustead, and Crawford needles, each with distinct design qualities to aid the process.
2. Epidural Catheter: The catheter enables for the continuous or intermittent injection of anesthetic drugs into the epidural space. It is normally built from flexible, biocompatible materials and may have varied tip configurations (e.g., open-ended, closed-ended with side holes).
3. Syringes: Syringes of varied sizes are supplied for the administration of local anesthetics, saline for loss of resistance method, and test dosages.
4. Filters: Filters are employed to avoid the entrance of particulate particles into the epidural space during injection.
5. Antiseptic Solutions: These solutions (e.g., chlorhexidine, iodine) are provided to prepare the skin and limit the risk of infection.
6. Curtains and Towels: Sterile curtains and towels assist maintain a sterile field throughout the process.
7. Local Anesthetics: Vials or ampoules of frequently used local anesthetics (e.g., lidocaine, bupivacaine) are supplied for initial and maintenance dosage.
8. Ancillary goods: Additional goods such as adhesive tape, sterile gloves, and marking pens may also be supplied to aid with the treatment.

Detailed Examination of Epidural Kit Components
Epidural Needles
The choice of epidural needle considerably determines the success of the surgery. The following sections give an in-depth look at the design and

function of the different kinds of needles included in epidural kits.

1. Tuohy Needle: The Tuohy needle, with its curved, blunt tip, is the most often used needle for epidural anesthesia. Its design sends the catheter into the epidural area, lowering the danger of dural puncture.
2. Hustead Needle: Similar to the Tuohy needle but with a less noticeable curvature, the Hustead needle provides an option for doctors depending on personal choice and unique procedural requirements.
3. Crawford Needle: The Crawford needle boasts a straight, thin-walled construction with a slight bevel, offering another choice for specific clinical settings.

The needles are available in various gauges (usually 16G to 18G) and lengths (8 to 18 cm) to fit diverse patient anatomies and procedure needs. Each needle is fitted with a stylet to prevent tissue or blood from blocking the lumen during insertion.

Epidural Catheters

Epidural catheters supplied in the kits are intended to administer anesthetic drugs efficiently into the epidural area. Key aspects of epidural catheters include:

1. Material: Made from flexible, biocompatible materials such as polyurethane or nylon, which balance flexibility and strength, enabling the catheter to transit the epidural area without kinking.
2. Lumens: Available in single or multiple lumens. Multi-lumen catheters allow for the simultaneous administration of multiple medications, boosting pain control capabilities.
3. Tip Design: The tip may be open-ended or closed-ended with several side holes. Open-ended catheters give a direct conduit for anesthetics, whereas closed-ended catheters with side holes allow a more dispersed administration.

Syringes

Syringes provided in epidural kits vary in size and are used for various reasons throughout the procedure:

1. 10 mL Syringes: Typically used for giving local anesthetics and saline for the loss of resistance method.
2. 5 mL Syringes: Often used for providing test doses to validate the catheter's insertion and verify there is no intravascular or intrathecal injection.
3. 1 mL Syringes: Used for accurate dosage and administration of lower quantities of anesthetic drugs or additives.

Filters

Filters are vital for ensuring that no particulate matter is introduced into the epidural area during injection. They assist preserve the sterility and safety of the surgery. Common kinds of filters included in epidural kits are:

1. 0.2 Micron Filters: Used to filter out germs and particulate debris from solutions before they are injected.
2. Bacterial Filters: Specifically developed to limit the entrance of germs into the epidural area, minimizing the risk of infection.

Antiseptic Solutions

Maintaining a sterile field is crucial in epidural anesthesia to avoid infections. Epidural kits often comprise antiseptic liquids such as:

1. Chlorhexidine: A frequently used antiseptic that has broad-spectrum antibacterial action. It is available in different concentrations (e.g., 0.5%, 2%) and formulations (e.g., aqueous, alcohol-based).
2. Povidone-Iodine: Another extensively used antiseptic, povidone-iodine has good antibacterial action and is available in different

concentrations.

Drapes and Towels

Sterile drapes and towels are crucial for maintaining a sterile field throughout the process. They are used to cover the patient and surrounding region, ensuring that only the prepared skin area is exposed.

1. Sterile curtains: Large curtains that cover the patient and the procedure area, preserving sterility.
2. Sterile Towels: Smaller towels used to isolate the injection site and give further protection against infection.

Local Anesthetics

Epidural kits frequently compromise vials or ampoules of widely used local anesthetics, such as:

1. Lidocaine: A fast-acting local anesthetic used for first dosages and test doses to confirm catheter insertion.
2. Bupivacaine: A longer-acting local anesthetic used for continuous infusion or intermittent boluses to sustain analgesia.

The concentration and amount of local anesthetics contained in the kits may vary depending on the intended application and clinical preferences.

Ancillary Items

Epidural kits also comprise several supplementary products that aid in the procedure:

1. Adhesive Tape: Used to keep the epidural catheter in place after implantation, guaranteeing stability and avoiding dislodgement.
2. Sterile Gloves: Essential for maintaining aseptic technique throughout

the process.
3. Marking Pens: Used to mark anatomical landmarks and aid needle insertion.

Principles and Techniques for Using Epidural Kits

The proper use of epidural kits demands a full grasp of the ideas and practices involved in each phase of the operation. The following sections highlight the essential ideas and recommended practices for utilizing epidural kits efficiently.

Preparation and Setup

1. Patient Preparation: Properly prepare the patient by situating them adequately (e.g., lateral decubitus or sitting posture) and identifying anatomical landmarks. Ensure the patient is informed about the surgery and has obtained consent.
2. Sterile Technique: Adhere to stringent sterile practices during the treatment. Use sterile gloves, drapes, and antiseptic solutions to prepare the injection site.
3. Kit Inspection: Inspect the contents of the epidural kit to verify all required components are present and sterile. Check the expiry dates of all items.

Needle Insertion and Identification of Epidural Space

1. Landmark Identification: Accurately identify anatomical landmarks (e.g., iliac crests, spinous processes) to establish the optimal insertion location.
2. Needle Insertion: Insert the epidural needle at a 90-degree angle to the skin with the bevel pointing cephalad. Advance the needle gently, utilizing the loss of resistance method or the hanging drop technique to find the epidural space.

3. Confirmation: Confirm the needle's location in the epidural space by noting a lack of resistance or a decrease in fluid level.

Catheter Insertion and Securing

1. Catheter Insertion: Gently insert the epidural catheter through the needle into the epidural space. Advance the catheter 3-5 cm beyond the needle tip to ensure it is properly positioned.
2. Resistance Check: Ensure little resistance when threading the catheter. If resistance is experienced, remove the catheter slightly and try to re-thread. Avoid straining the catheter to avoid kinking or injury.
3. Needle Removal: Once the catheter is in place, gently extract the needle while maintaining the catheter steady. Ensure the catheter stays in place during needle removal.
4. Securing the Catheter: Secure the catheter with adhesive tape and sterile dressing to avoid dislodgement. Use additional fastening techniques, such as tunneling or adhesive anchors, if required.

Administration and Monitoring

1. Initial Test Dose: Administer an initial test dose of local anesthetic to check catheter insertion and rule out intravascular or intrathecal injection. Monitor the patient for any symptoms of toxicity or adverse reactions.
2. Continuous Infusion or Intermittent Boluses: Depending on the clinical circumstances, deliver continuous infusion or intermittent boluses of local anesthetic via the catheter. Adjust the dose depending on the patient's reaction and amount of analgesia necessary.
3. Monitoring: Continuously monitor the patient for indicators of effective analgesia, possible problems, and general well-being. Adjust the infusion rate or bolus dose as required to ensure optimum pain

management.

Advanced Techniques and Considerations

The usage of epidural kits may include sophisticated procedures and considerations to optimize the safety and effectiveness of the treatment. The next sections address some of these sophisticated elements.

Ultrasound Guidance

Ultrasound guidance has become an increasingly helpful technique in the insertion of epidural needles and catheters, especially in patients with complicated anatomy or problematic landmarks.

1. view: Ultrasound offers real-time view of the needle route, epidural space, and surrounding structures, enhancing accuracy and minimizing the risk of complications.
2. Technique: Use ultrasonography to locate the ideal insertion location, guide needle advancement, and confirm catheter implantation. This approach may be especially effective in obese individuals or those with abnormal spinal architecture.

Combined Spinal-Epidural (CSE) Technique

The combined spinal-epidural (CSE) approach combines the advantages of both spinal and epidural anesthesia, giving quick onset of analgesia with the flexibility of prolonged pain management.

1. Procedure: Perform the first spinal injection with a spinal needle placed via the epidural needle, followed by the installation of the epidural catheter for continuous analgesia.
2. Benefits: The CSE procedure delivers immediate onset of pain relief from the spinal injection and lasting analgesia from the epidural catheter. It is widely used in obstetric anesthetic and some surgical

operations.

Patient-Specific Considerations

Tailoring the usage of epidural kits to individual patient features and clinical circumstances is critical for optimal results. Consider the following patient-specific factors:

1. Anatomical Variations: Adjust the choice of needle and catheter length depending on the patient's body habitus and anatomical landmarks. Use ultrasound guidance as required.
2. Coexisting disorders: Consider any coexisting medical disorders (e.g., coagulopathy, spinal anomalies) that may impair the surgery and need adjustments to the method or equipment.
3. Patient Preferences: Take into consideration the patient's preferences and concerns, offering clear explanations and resolving any questions or anxiety.

Innovations in Epidural Kits

Ongoing breakthroughs in technology and materials science continue to drive improvements in epidural kits, boosting their safety, effectiveness, and user-friendliness. Some important inventions include:

1. Echogenic Needles: Echogenic needles with greater visibility under ultrasound guidance improve the precision of needle placement and lower the risk of complications.
2. Integrated Catheter Systems: Advanced catheter systems with integrated sensors and feedback mechanisms give real-time data on catheter placement and performance, boosting safety and effectiveness.
3. Improved Materials: Innovations in materials research have led to the creation of more flexible, biocompatible, and durable catheters, enhancing patient comfort and minimizing the risk of problems.

Conclusion

The full knowledge and proper use of epidural kits are important to the successful delivery of lumbar epidural anesthesia. By knowing the components, concepts, and advanced procedures related with epidural kits, doctors may increase the safety, efficiency, and efficacy of the process. Continuous education, clinical practice, and innovation in equipment design will further develop the discipline, assuring best results for patients having lumbar epidural anesthesia. Through attentive application of these concepts and approaches, healthcare personnel may give high-quality treatment and effective pain management in a range of clinical settings.

7.3. Monitoring Equipment

In the field of anesthesia, careful monitoring is as crucial as the delivery of anesthetic medications. Monitoring equipment acts as the clinician's eyes and ears, delivering real-time data on the patient's physiological status during lumbar epidural anesthesia. This chapter digs into the full specifics of monitoring equipment utilized in this context, studying the many kinds of monitors, their unique roles, and the concepts underlying their functioning. By learning the use and interpretation of monitoring technology, doctors may increase patient safety, optimize anesthetic administration, and rapidly treat any issues that may emerge.

Importance of Monitoring in Lumbar Epidural Anesthesia

Monitoring is vital in anesthesia to guarantee patient safety and the successful control of the anesthetic procedure. It comprises continuous measurement of vital signs and physiological data, allowing quick treatments and modifications. The major aims of monitoring during lumbar epidural anesthesia include:

1. Maintaining Hemodynamic Stability: Monitoring aids in recognizing and treating changes in blood pressure, heart rate, and cardiac output.

2. Ensuring Adequate Oxygenation and Ventilation: Continuous evaluation of respiratory parameters ensures the patient is appropriately oxygenated and ventilated.
3. Detecting Complications Early: Real-time monitoring enables for the early diagnosis of complications such as hypotension, bradycardia, respiratory depression, and neurological disorders.
4. Guiding Anesthetic maintenance: Monitoring data directs the modification of anesthetic medication doses and the maintenance of the epidural catheter.
5. Enhancing Patient Safety: By delivering continuous data, monitoring equipment promotes overall patient safety and improves results.

Types of Monitoring Equipment

Several kinds of monitoring devices are deployed during lumbar epidural anesthesia, each having a distinct function. The major types of monitoring equipment include:

1. Cardiovascular Monitors
2. Respiratory Monitors
3. Neuromuscular Monitors
4. Temperature Monitors
5. Miscellaneous Monitors
6. Cardiovascular Monitors: Cardiovascular monitors are crucial for measuring the patient's heart function and circulation state. Key kinds of cardiovascular monitoring include:

- Electrocardiogram (ECG)
- Non-invasive Blood Pressure (NIBP) Monitors
- Invasive Blood Pressure (IBP) Monitors
- Pulse Oximetry
- Cardiac Output Monitors
- Electrocardiogram (ECG)

The ECG is a vital tool for monitoring heart rate and rhythm. It enables real-time tracking of the electrical activity of the heart, assisting in the diagnosis of arrhythmias, myocardial ischemia, and other cardiac diseases.

- Components: ECG monitoring comprises electrodes put on the patient's chest and limbs, coupled to a monitor that shows the heart's electrical activity.
- Function: The ECG records the heart's electrical impulses, generating a graphical depiction (P, QRS, and T waves) that doctors can interpret.
- Clinical Relevance: Continuous ECG monitoring during epidural anesthesia is critical for identifying arrhythmias, myocardial ischemia, and other cardiac abnormalities.
- Non-invasive Blood Pressure (NIBP) Monitors

NIBP monitors offer frequent readings of blood pressure utilizing a cuff and an automated inflation/deflation mechanism.

1. Components: NIBP monitors consist of an inflated cuff, a pressure sensor, and a monitor showing the systolic, diastolic, and mean arterial pressure.
2. Function: The cuff inflates to occlude blood flow, then gently deflates as the monitor detects oscillations in the artery to determine blood pressure.
3. Clinical Relevance: Regular blood pressure monitoring is necessary to identify hypotension or hypertension during epidural anesthesia, allowing for prompt management.

- **Invasive Blood Pressure (IBP) Monitors**

IBP monitors use the direct monitoring of arterial pressure with an arterial catheter, delivering continuous and reliable blood pressure readings.

- Components: IBP monitoring needs an arterial catheter, a pressure

transducer, and a monitor showing the arterial pressure waveform.
- Function: The arterial catheter sends pressure changes to the transducer, which transforms them into electrical impulses presented as a continuous waveform.
- Clinical Relevance: IBP monitoring is especially effective in high-risk patients or complicated operations where continuous and accurate blood pressure monitoring is needed.
- Pulse Oximetry

Pulse oximetry analyzes the oxygen saturation of hemoglobin in the blood, giving a non-invasive approach to monitor oxygenation.

- Components: Pulse oximeters employ a probe connected to a finger, earlobe, or toe, and a monitor showing oxygen saturation (SpO2) and pulse rate.
- Function: The probe produces light at two wavelengths, which is absorbed differentially by oxygenated and deoxygenated hemoglobin. The monitor determines SpO2 based on the absorption differences.
- Clinical Relevance: Continuous monitoring of oxygen saturation is crucial to provide sufficient oxygenation, diagnose hypoxemia early, and guide oxygen treatment.
- Cardiac Output Monitors

Cardiac output monitors assess the amount of blood the heart pumps every minute, giving significant information regarding cardiac function and hemodynamic health.

- Types: Various techniques exist, including thermodilution, pulse contour analysis, and bioimpedance.
- Function: Each approach utilizes distinct concepts to assess cardiac output. For example, thermodilution involves injecting a cold saline bolus into the central circulation and detecting temperature changes downstream.

- Clinical Relevance: Monitoring cardiac output aids in monitoring the heart's pumping efficiency and directing fluid and vasoactive medication management.

2. Respiratory Monitors

Respiratory monitors are vital for measuring and providing proper breathing and oxygenation. Key kinds of respiratory monitors include:

1. Capnography
2. Spirometry
3. Respiratory Rate Monitors

- Capnography

Capnography detects the concentration of carbon dioxide (CO_2) in exhaled air, giving real-time data on ventilation.

- Components: Capnographs consist of a sampling line attached to the patient's airway and a monitor showing the CO_2 concentration as a waveform (capnogram).
- Function: The capnograph detects the CO_2 concentration during the respiratory cycle, generating a waveform that indicates the patient's ventilation status.
- Clinical Relevance: Capnography is vital for recognizing hypoventilation, apnea, and airway obstruction, as well as directing modifications in ventilatory support.
- Spirometry

Spirometry assesses lung function by monitoring the volume and flow of air during intake and exhalation.

- Components: Spirometers feature a mouthpiece coupled to a flow sensor and a monitor showing spirometric data such as tidal volume,

vital capacity, and forced expiratory volume.
- Function: The spirometer measures the volume and flow of air during breathing movements, giving data on lung function and respiratory mechanics.
- Clinical Relevance: Spirometry is important for testing respiratory function preoperatively, monitoring changes during anesthesia, and evaluating lung function in patients with respiratory diseases.
- Respiratory Rate Monitors

Respiratory rate monitors allow continuous monitoring of the patient's respiratory rate.

- Components: These monitors employ sensors inserted on the chest or belly to detect breathing movements, with the rate shown on a monitor.
- Function: The sensors detect the rise and fall of the chest or belly while breathing, computing the respiratory rate.
- Clinical Relevance: Continuous monitoring of respiratory rate is critical for recognizing respiratory depression or apnea, especially in patients taking sedative or narcotic drugs.

3. Neuromuscular Monitors

Neuromuscular monitors measure the function of neuromuscular transmission, especially in patients receiving neuromuscular blocking drugs.

1. Train-of-Four (TOF) Monitors
2. Peripheral Nerve Stimulators

- Train-of-Four (TOF) Monitors

TOF monitors measure neuromuscular function by applying a series of electrical stimulation to a peripheral nerve and detecting the subsequent muscle contractions.

- Components: TOF monitors comprise of a nerve stimulator, electrodes placed over a peripheral nerve (e.g., ulnar, face), and a monitor showing the contraction response.
- Function: The nerve stimulator administers four electrical pulses in fast succession, and the monitor evaluates the muscle reaction, giving data on the degree of neuromuscular blockade.
- Clinical Relevance: TOF monitoring is critical for measuring the degree of neuromuscular blockade, directing the dose of neuromuscular blocking medications, and ensuring appropriate recovery before extubation.
- Peripheral Nerve Stimulators

Peripheral nerve stimulators are used to measure neuromuscular function by providing electrical stimulation to a peripheral nerve and measuring the muscle response.

- Components: Nerve stimulators contain a portable device with electrodes that send electrical pulses to a peripheral nerve.
- Function: The stimulator administers a regulated electrical stimulation, and the doctor watches the ensuing muscle contraction to measure neuromuscular function.
- Clinical Relevance: Peripheral nerve stimulation is beneficial for monitoring neuromuscular blockade and directing the dose of neuromuscular blocking medications during anesthesia.

4. Temperature Monitors

Temperature monitoring are necessary for preserving normothermia during anesthesia, since hypothermia may lead to serious problems.

1. Core Temperature Monitors
2. Skin Temperature Monitors

- Core Temperature Monitors

Core temperature monitors measure the patient's interior body temperature, giving a precise evaluation of thermal state.

- Types: Common techniques include esophageal probes, tympanic membrane thermometers, and bladder or rectal thermometers.
- Function: These monitors detect temperature in key body sites, reflecting the patient's core temperature.
- Clinical Relevance: Maintaining normothermia is critical for minimizing perioperative problems such as surgical site infections, coagulopathies, and delayed recovery. Core temperature monitoring helps doctors discover and manage deviations from the intended temperature range immediately.
- Skin Temperature Monitors

Skin temperature monitors analyze the temperature of the patient's skin surface, giving extra information on thermal state.

- Types: Skin temperature may be monitored using infrared thermometers, surface probes, or thermal imaging systems.
- Function: These monitors measure temperature variations on the skin's surface, which may suggest peripheral vasoconstriction or vasodilation.
- Clinical Relevance: Skin temperature monitoring complements core temperature monitoring and assists in measuring peripheral perfusion and thermal comfort.

5. Miscellaneous Monitors

Miscellaneous monitors cover a number of specialized devices used to monitor certain parameters or physiological processes under anesthesia.

1. Depth of Anesthesia Monitors
2. Cerebral Oximetry Monitors
3. Bispectral Index (BIS) Monitors

- Depth of Anesthesia Monitors

Depth of anesthesia monitors analyze the patient's degree of awareness and anesthetic depth using different physiological markers and algorithms.

- Types: These monitors may employ electroencephalography (EEG), processed EEG (pEEG), or other modalities to assess the patient's degree of awareness.
- Function: Depth of anesthesia monitors examine EEG signals or other data to generate a numerical number indicating the patient's anesthetic depth.
- Clinical Relevance: Monitoring the depth of anesthesia aids in titrating anesthetic medications to obtain the appropriate amount of unconsciousness while reducing the danger of awareness or excessive sedation.
- Cerebral Oximetry Monitors

Cerebral oximetry monitors assess regional cerebral oxygen saturation (rSO2), offering insights on brain perfusion and oxygenation.

- Components: These monitors employ near-infrared spectroscopy (NIRS) to evaluate oxygen saturation in the brain tissue.
- Function: Cerebral oximetry monitors send near-infrared light into the scalp, which penetrates the underlying tissues and is absorbed by hemoglobin. The reflected light is examined to determine rSO2.
- Clinical Relevance: Monitoring cerebral oxygenation assists in diagnosing cerebral hypoperfusion and directing therapies to improve cerebral perfusion pressure.
- Bispectral Index (BIS) Monitors

BIS monitors measure the patient's degree of awareness and sedation based on EEG readings and signal processing algorithms.

- Components: BIS monitors employ EEG electrodes placed on the

patient's forehead to measure and analyze brainwave patterns.
- Function: Signal processing techniques translate EEG data into a numerical value (BIS score) reflecting the patient's degree of awareness, with lower scores indicating deeper anesthesia.
- Clinical Relevance: BIS monitoring supports doctors in titrating anesthetic drugs to maintain the optimum degree of sedation while limiting the danger of intraoperative consciousness and encouraging speedy recovery.

6. Principles of Monitoring Equipment Use

The proper use of monitoring equipment involves adherence to specific principles and best practices to enable reliable data gathering and interpretation.

1. Proper Placement: Ensure that sensors, electrodes, and probes are accurately positioned to produce reliable data.
2. Calibration: Regularly calibrate monitoring equipment to ensure accuracy and dependability.
3. Baseline Assessment: Establish baseline values for each monitored parameter before the initiation of anesthesia to simplify interpretation of changes.
4. Continuous Monitoring: Maintain continuous monitoring during the anesthetic procedure to notice changes swiftly.
5. Integration: Integrate data from numerous monitors to get a full evaluation of the patient's physiological condition.
6. Alarm Thresholds: Set suitable alarm thresholds for monitored metrics to trigger prompt interventions when irregularities occur.
7. Documentation: Document all monitoring data correctly and extensively in the patient's medical record for future reference and analysis.

Advanced Monitoring Techniques and Innovations

Advancements in monitoring technology continue to expand the capabilities and accuracy of monitoring systems. Some important advances and approaches include:

1. Artificial Intelligence (AI): Integration of AI algorithms with monitoring systems for real-time data analysis and predictive analytics.
2. Remote Monitoring: Wireless and telemedicine-enabled monitoring systems that allow for remote data gathering and analysis, providing continuous observation and early intervention.
3. Multimodal Monitoring: Integration of numerous monitoring modalities (e.g., EEG, NIRS, ECG) onto a single platform to offer a thorough evaluation of the patient's physiological condition.
4. Smart alerts: Intelligent alarm systems that prioritize alerts based on clinical importance and alter alarm levels dynamically to avoid false alarms.
5. Miniaturization: Development of tiny, portable monitoring equipment that promote mobility and flexibility in diverse therapeutic situations.

Conclusion

Monitoring equipment serves a significant role in guaranteeing the safety and effectiveness of lumbar epidural anesthesia by giving real-time data on the patient's physiological condition. By knowing the fundamentals of monitoring equipment utilization, doctors may optimize anesthetic administration, discover issues early, and enhance patient outcomes. Continued improvements in monitoring technology show promise for further strengthening the capabilities and accuracy of monitoring devices, opening the path for safer and more effective anesthetic treatment. Through continual education, training, and research, healthcare practitioners may remain ahead of the newest innovations in monitoring devices and apply them into clinical practice efficiently.

Chapter 8

COMPLICATIONS AND MANAGEMENT

8.1 Immediate Complications

Administering lumbar epidural anesthesia is a complicated surgery that demands cautious skill and an in-depth awareness of possible problems. Immediate problems might emerge during or shortly after the treatment, typically demanding rapid detection and intervention to reduce severe consequences. This section will cover the many acute problems related with lumbar epidural anesthesia, their etiology, clinical presentation, and options for efficient therapy.

Types of Immediate Complications

Immediate consequences from lumbar epidural anesthesia may essentially be categorized into numerous categories:

1. Cardiovascular Complications
2. Respiratory Complications
3. Neurological Complications
4. Infectious Complications
5. Technical Complications

- Cardiovascular Complications

- Cardiovascular problems are among the most prevalent acute adverse effects linked with lumbar epidural anesthesia. They might vary from moderate hypotension to catastrophic cardiac problems.

Hypotension

Hypotension is a prevalent consequence after lumbar epidural anesthesia due to the sympathetic blocking that leads to vasodilation and reduced venous return.

1. Pathophysiology: The anesthetic drug inhibits sympathetic nerves, resulting in vasodilation, decreased venous return, and reduced cardiac output.
2. Clinical Presentation: Symptoms may include dizziness, light-headedness, nausea, and in extreme instances, loss of consciousness.
3. Care: Initial care comprises placing the patient in a left lateral or Trendelenburg position, delivering intravenous fluids to enhance preload, and utilizing vasopressors such ephedrine or phenylephrine to counteract vasodilation.

Bradycardia

Bradycardia may develop owing to the blockage of cardiac accelerator fibers (T1-T4) or as a reflex reaction to reduced venous return.

1. Pathophysiology: The sympathetic blockade decreases heart rate and cardiac output, possibly leading to bradycardia.
2. Clinical Presentation: Patients may appear with a sluggish heart rate, hypotension, dizziness, or syncope.
3. Management: Management involves atropine injection to raise heart rate, epinephrine in severe instances, and providing proper volume status using intravenous fluids.

Cardiac Arrest

Though uncommon, cardiac arrest may occur and demands prompt attention.

1. Pathophysiology: Severe hypotension and bradycardia may escalate to cardiac arrest if not handled immediately.
2. Clinical Presentation: Absence of pulse, unresponsiveness, and apnea are characteristic findings.
3. Management: Immediate cardiac resuscitation (CPR) following Advanced Cardiovascular Life Support (ACLS) procedures is needed. Epinephrine and other emergency drugs should be supplied, and the underlying cause (e.g., severe hypotension) should be immediately treated.

Respiratory Complications

Respiratory problems, albeit less prevalent, may be life-threatening and need rapid care.

Respiratory Depression

Respiratory depression may develop from excessive spinal anesthesia or the use of opioid adjuncts.

1. Pathophysiology: Anesthetic drugs or opioids may depress the respiratory centers in the brainstem or create excessive spinal blockage affecting the respiratory muscles.
2. Clinical Presentation: Symptoms include slow and shallow breathing, reduced oxygen saturation, and in extreme instances, respiratory arrest.
3. Management: Supportive interventions include supplementary oxygen, airway management using bag-valve-mask ventilation, and the use of naloxone for opioid-induced respiratory depression.

Pneumothorax

Although uncommon, pneumothorax may develop if the needle punctures the pleura during the epidural surgery.

1. Pathophysiology: Accidental penetration of the pleura leads to the entry of air into the pleural cavity, causing lung collapse.
2. Clinical Presentation: Symptoms include abrupt chest discomfort, dyspnea, and reduced breath sounds on the afflicted side.
3. Treatment: Immediate treatment comprises oxygen delivery and chest tube insertion to re-expand the lung.

Neurological Complications

Neurological consequences might vary from temporary symptoms to lifelong abnormalities, demanding attentive monitoring and management.

Post-Dural Puncture Headache (PDPH)

PDPH is a frequent complication occurring from unintentional dural puncture.

1. Pathophysiology: Leakage of cerebrospinal fluid (CSF) from the puncture site leads to reduced CSF pressure, producing headache.
2. Clinical Presentation: Headache increases in an upright posture and improves after laying down. It may be accompanied by nausea, photophobia, and neck stiffness.
3. Treatment: Initial treatment involves bed rest, water, and caffeine. If symptoms continue, an epidural blood patch may be applied to seal the dural puncture.

Nerve Injury

Direct needle trauma or ischemia may result in nerve damage, appearing with motor or sensory impairments.

1. Pathophysiology: Needle trauma or compression from hematoma

development may injure nerve fibers.
2. Clinical Presentation: Symptoms include numbness, tingling, motor weakness, or intense pain in the affected limb.
3. Management: Immediate stop of the surgery, neurological examination, and imaging procedures (e.g., MRI) to determine the degree of the damage. Surgical consultation may be necessary for hematoma evacuation or nerve repair.

Infectious Complications

Infectious problems, albeit less prevalent, may be dangerous and need rapid diagnosis and treatment.

Epidural Abscess

An epidural abscess might develop owing to bacterial contamination during the treatment.

1. Pathophysiology: Introduction of microorganisms into the epidural region might lead to localized infection and abscess development.
2. Clinical Presentation: Symptoms include severe back pain, fever, and neurological abnormalities such as radiculopathy or myelopathy.
3. Management: Immediate delivery of broad-spectrum antibiotics and surgical draining of the abscess if required.

Technical Complications

Technical issues originate from challenges encountered during the treatment itself.

Intravascular Injection

Accidental intravascular injection of the anesthetic agent may lead to systemic toxicity.

1. Pathophysiology: Inadvertent injection into a blood artery leads to high plasma levels of the anesthetic, generating systemic effects.

2. Clinical Presentation: Symptoms include tinnitus, metallic taste, perioral numbness, convulsions, and cardiovascular collapse.
3. Management: Immediate withdrawal of injection, delivery of lipid emulsion treatment, and supportive care including airway management and seizure control.

High Spinal Anesthesia

High spinal anesthesia may develop if the anesthetic extends cephalad, impacting the thoracic and cervical areas.

1. Pathophysiology: Excessive distribution of the anesthetic drug might result in excessive spinal blockage, compromising cardiac and respiratory function.
2. Clinical Presentation: Symptoms include hypotension, bradycardia, respiratory distress, and altered mental state.
3. Management: Supportive interventions include placing the patient with a head-down tilt, providing intravenous fluids, vasopressors, and maintaining sufficient breathing.

8.2 Delayed Complications

Delayed problems may emerge hours to days after the application of lumbar epidural anesthesia. These problems need constant observation and prompt action to avoid long-term consequences.

Types of Delayed Complications

Delayed complications include:

1. Infectious Complications
2. Neurological Complications
3. Hematological Complications
4. Chronic Pain Syndromes

- Infectious Complications

Delayed infectious consequences might develop as localized or systemic illnesses.

Epidural Abscess

An epidural abscess might manifest days to weeks post-procedure, necessitating strong clinical suspicion for diagnosis.

1. Pathophysiology: Persistent or delayed bacterial infection might lead to abscess development.
2. Clinical Presentation: Symptoms include back discomfort, fever, and increasing neurological impairments.
3. Management: Prolonged antibiotic treatment and surgical drainage are typically necessary.

Meningitis

Meningitis is a dangerous consequence occurring from the spread of infection to the meninges.

1. Pathophysiology: Bacterial or viral pathogens introduced during the surgery may infect the meninges.
2. Clinical Presentation: Symptoms include headache, neck stiffness, fever, photophobia, and impaired mental state.
3. Management: Empirical antibiotic treatment began promptly, followed by customized therapy based on culture findings. Supportive treatment in an intensive care unit may be essential for severe instances.

Neurological Complications

Neurological problems might appear days to weeks following the treatment, presenting with a variety of symptoms.

Arachnoiditis

Arachnoiditis is an inflammatory disorder of the arachnoid membrane, which may emerge as a delayed consequence.

1. Pathophysiology: Inflammation of the arachnoid membrane may develop from chemical irritation, infection, or surgical damage.
2. Clinical Presentation: Symptoms include severe back pain, scorching agony in the lower limbs, and neurological abnormalities such as paralysis or sensory loss.
3. Management: Treatment comprises the use of corticosteroids to decrease inflammation, pain management methods, and physical therapy. In extreme circumstances, surgical intervention may be necessary.

Chronic Radiculopathy

Chronic radiculopathy may occur owing to prolonged nerve root irritation or damage.

1. Pathophysiology: Prolonged nerve root compression or irritation leads to persistent pain and neurological impairments.
2. Clinical Presentation: Symptoms include chronic back discomfort, radiating pain along the damaged nerve root, and motor or sensory impairments.
3. Control: Management involves pain control with drugs, epidural steroid injections, physical therapy, and in refractory situations, surgical intervention.

Hematological Complications

Hematological problems, such as epidural hematoma, might appear as delayed consequences, typically needing surgical intervention.

Epidural Hematoma

An epidural hematoma may form owing to bleeding into the epidural space, presenting with delayed start of symptoms.

1. Pathophysiology: Traumatic needle insertion or anticoagulant treatment might cause bleeding and hematoma development.
2. Clinical Presentation: Symptoms include severe back pain, neurologi-

cal impairments, and bowel or bladder problems.
3. Management: Urgent MRI to assess the extent of the hematoma, followed by surgical evacuation to decompress the spinal cord.

Chronic Pain Syndromes
Chronic pain syndromes may arise as a consequence of nerve injury or prolonged inflammation.

Complex Regional Pain Syndrome (CRPS)
CRPS is a persistent pain disease that may occur after nerve damage or trauma.

1. Pathophysiology: Abnormal reaction of the peripheral and central nervous systems to nerve damage or trauma.
2. Clinical Presentation: Symptoms include severe, prolonged pain, edema, changes in skin color and temperature, and motor dysfunction.
3. Management: Multimodal treatment involving pain medicines, physical therapy, sympathetic nerve blocks, and psychological support.

8.3 Management and Treatment Strategies

Effective management and treatment of problems related with lumbar epidural anesthesia need a complete strategy, including prevention, early identification, and appropriate intervention.

Preventive Strategies
Preventive techniques are critical in lowering the risk of problems during lumbar epidural anesthesia.

Patient Assessment and Preparation
Thorough preoperative examination and preparation are needed to identify individuals at greater risk of problems.

1. Medical History: Review the patient's medical history, including any history of cardiovascular, respiratory, or neurological issues.
2. Physical Examination: Conduct a complete physical examination concentrating on the spine and neurological function.
3. Laboratory Tests: Perform essential laboratory tests, including coagulation studies, to determine the patient's fitness for the surgery.
4. Patient Education: Educate the patient about the surgery, its hazards, and postoperative care to achieve informed consent and compliance.

Aseptic Technique
Adhering to proper aseptic practices is crucial to avoid infection problems.

1. Hand Hygiene: Ensure complete handwashing and use of sterile gloves.
2. Sterile Field: Maintain a sterile field throughout the process, employing sterile drapes, equipment, and solutions.
3. Skin Preparation: Prepare the skin with antiseptic treatments such as chlorhexidine or povidone-iodine.

Technique and Equipment
Using suitable procedures and equipment may lessen the chance of technical problems.

1. Needle Insertion: Use suitable needle sizes and procedures to reduce tissue stress and the danger of dural puncture.
2. Epidural Space Identification: Employ methods such as the lack of resistance to air or saline to precisely identify the epidural space.
3. Monitoring: Continuously monitor the patient's vital signs throughout the operation to discover and manage any urgent issues immediately.

Early Detection and Intervention
Early diagnosis and response are crucial to treating problems efficiently.
Monitoring
Continuous monitoring of the patient's vital signs and neurological

condition throughout and after the surgery is crucial.

1. Cardiovascular Monitoring: Monitor blood pressure, heart rate, and oxygen saturation continually.
2. Breathing Monitoring: Assess breathing rate, oxygenation, and symptoms of respiratory distress.
3. Neurological Monitoring: Evaluate the patient's motor and sensory function periodically to discover any neurological abnormalities early.

Prompt Intervention

Timely management may prevent issues from worsening and improve patient outcomes.

1. Hypotension Management: Administer intravenous fluids and vasopressors rapidly to address hypotension.
2. Bradycardia Management: Use atropine or epinephrine to treat severe bradycardia.
3. Respiratory Support: Provide supplementary oxygen and ventilatory support as required to alleviate respiratory depression.
4. Neurological evaluation: Perform a complete neurological evaluation to discover and correct any nerve damage or impairments quickly.

Treatment Strategies for Specific Complications

Effective treatment options customized to individual issues are crucial for improved patient outcomes.

Infectious Complications

1. Antibiotic treatment: Initiate broad-spectrum antibiotics quickly for suspected infections, customizing treatment depending on culture findings.
2. Surgical Intervention: Surgical drainage may be essential for abscesses or severe infections.

CHAPTER 8

Neurological Complications

1. Pain Management: Use analgesics, anti-inflammatory medications, and nerve blocks to control pain associated with nerve injury.
2. Physical Therapy: Implement physical therapy to enhance motor function and avoid long-term impairment.
3. Surgical Intervention: Surgical decompression may be necessary for severe instances of nerve damage or epidural hematoma.

Hematological Complications

1. Imaging Studies: Perform MRI or CT scans to determine the extent of hematomas.
2. Surgical Evacuation: Surgical evacuation of hematomas is important to reduce spinal cord compression and avoid lasting impairments.

Rehabilitation and Long-term Care

Rehabilitation and long-term care are necessary for individuals recovering from consequences of lumbar epidural anesthesia.

Pain Management

Chronic pain treatment demands a multimodal strategy to enhance patient quality of life.

1. Treatments: Use a mixture of analgesics, anti-inflammatory meds, and neuropathic pain treatments.
2. Interventional Procedures: Consider epidural steroid injections, nerve blocks, or spinal cord stimulation for refractory pain.

Physical Rehabilitation

Physical rehabilitation strives to restore function and mobility.

1. Physical Therapy: Engage patients in physical therapy to increase strength, flexibility, and motor function.
2. Occupational Therapy: Occupational therapy may assist patients recover independence in everyday tasks.

Psychological Support

Psychological assistance is vital for people suffering with chronic pain and impairment.

1. Therapy: Provide therapy to assist patients deal with pain and emotional anguish.
2. Support Groups: Encourage involvement in support groups for patients with comparable disorders.

Conclusion

Managing problems related with lumbar epidural anesthesia needs a comprehensive strategy that includes prevention, early identification, immediate management, and long-term care. By following best practices, adopting suitable procedures, and implementing effective treatment strategies, doctors may limit the risk of problems and optimize patient outcomes. Continuous education, training, and adherence to evidence-based recommendations are critical for sustaining good standards of care in the administration of lumbar epidural anesthesia.

Chapter 9

EPIDURAL ANESTHESIA IN SPECIAL POPULATIONS

Introduction

It is necessary to make certain adjustments while administering epidural anesthesia to certain populations in order to effectively control pain during surgical and obstetric operations. To guarantee safety and efficacy, individualized approaches are required for pediatric, geriatric, and pregnant patients due to their distinct anatomical, physiological, and pharmacological characteristics. Detailed evaluation, accurate medication dosage, careful technique, and close monitoring are the tenets of this chapter as it explores the complexities of administering epidural anesthesia to these varied populations.

9.1 Patients aged 0–17
Anatomical and Physiological Considerations

Administering epidural anesthesia in pediatric patients involves a grasp of their particular anatomical and physiological features. Children are more than just "small adults"; there are a number of important distinctions that cause their bodies to react differently to anesthesia:

Decreased Perioperative Area

1. Quantity: Compared to adults, children have a smaller and more pliable

epidural space. To obtain effective anesthesia without systemic toxicity, accurate dose is required since this affects the volume and dispersion of local anesthetics.
2. Variations in Development: The contents of the epidural space, such as fat and vascular, change as a kid develops, which affects the dynamics and pharmacokinetics of anesthetics.

The Nerve Fiber Density Is Greater

1. Increased Sensitivity: The larger density of nerve fibers in the juvenile population needs lower dosages of anesthetics to achieve the desired block.
2. Rapid Onset: The anesthetic effect sometimes comes more swiftly in youngsters owing to the heightened sensitivity of their neurological system.

Increased Cardiac Output

1. Systemic Absorption: Pediatric patients often have increased cardiac output, which may contribute to rapid systemic absorption of local anesthetics, raising the risk of toxicity if dose is not adequately regulated.

Drug Dosing and Selection

Choosing the right local anesthetic and dosage is crucial in pediatric epidural anesthesia. The selection is based on the patient's age, weight, and the desired duration and depth of anesthesia.

Bupivacaine

1. Usage: Bupivacaine is favored for its long duration of action and reliable safety profile.
2. Dosing: Typical concentrations range from 0.25% to 0.5%, with dosing

calculated based on weight (mg/kg) to ensure effective anesthesia while minimizing toxicity.

Ropivacaine

1. Advantages: Ropivacaine is preferred for its reduced cardiotoxicity and lower incidence of motor blockade, making it safer for prolonged procedures.
2. Dosing: Similar to bupivacaine, with modifications made per kilogram of body weight.

Lidocaine

1. Shorter operations: Lidocaine is beneficial for shorter operations because to its fast onset and intermediate duration.
2. Dosing: Typically approximately 1-2 mg/kg, with cautious titration to minimize systemic toxicity.

Needle and Catheter Selection

The choice of needle and catheter size is critical to avoid stress and guarantee correct insertion in young patients.

Needles

1. Size: Smaller gauge needles (22-25 gauge) are suggested to avoid tissue damage and permit simpler insertion.
2. Approach: The approach must be soft and accurate to prevent harm to the fragile tissues of the juvenile spine.

Catheters

1. Flexibility: Flexible, soft-tipped catheters are used to lessen the danger of nerve injury and permit easier insertion and placement.

2. Length: Catheter length should be adequate for the child's size to promote effective anesthetic while limiting the risk of problems.

Monitoring and Safety

Vigilant monitoring before and after the administration of epidural anesthesia is vital to identify any issues early and guarantee patient safety.

Vital Signs

1. Continuous Monitoring: Heart rate, blood pressure, and oxygen saturation should be continually monitored to identify any immediate adverse effects.
2. Baselines: Establishing baseline readings pre-procedure assists in recognizing substantial variations post-procedure.

Neurological Assessment

1. Sensory and Motor Function: Regular examination of sensory and motor function is required to achieve the optimal degree of anesthesia and identify any symptoms of neurotoxicity.
2. Age-Appropriate instruments: Use age-appropriate instruments and scales to measure pain and neurological function in pediatric patients.

Respiratory Monitoring

1. Respiratory Rate and Effort: Close monitoring of respiratory rate and effort, particularly in younger patients, is critical to identify early symptoms of respiratory depression.
2. Oxygenation: Supplemental oxygen should be readily accessible, and oxygen saturation measured continually.

Complications and Management

Complications with pediatric epidural anesthesia might include hypotension, bradycardia, and respiratory depression. Prompt detection and treatment are critical to maintain patient safety.

Hypotension

1. Management: Hypotension may be controlled by fluid boluses (e.g., crystalloids) and, if required, vasopressors. Monitoring for indicators of fluid excess is critical.

Bradycardia

1. Intervention: Severe bradycardia may be addressed with atropine, which raises heart rate by blocking the vagus nerve.

Respiratory Depression

1. Supportive Care: Respiratory depression may need supplementary oxygen and, in severe instances, assisted breathing. The anesthesia should be discontinued or lowered if respiratory depression is noted.

Special Considerations for Neonates and Infants

Neonates and newborns constitute a particularly susceptible segment within the pediatric population.

Immature Organ Systems

1. Liver and Kidney Function: Immature liver and kidney function in newborns and babies impacts the metabolism and excretion of anesthetics, requiring lower dosages and careful monitoring.
2. Central Nervous System: The growing CNS is more vulnerable to anesthetic effects, increasing the risk of neurotoxicity.

Blood-Brain Barrier

1. Permeability: The blood-brain barrier is more permeable in newborns, increasing the risk of central nervous system toxicity from local anesthetics.
2. Modified Dosing: Doses must be modified to account for the increased sensitivity and permeability of the blood-brain barrier.

Thermoregulation

1. Temperature Control: Neonates and babies are prone to hypothermia owing to their increased body surface area to weight ratio and undeveloped thermoregulatory systems.
2. Warming Devices: Use of warming devices and keeping a warm atmosphere is necessary during and after the process.

9.2 Geriatric Patients

Anatomical and Physiological Changes

Geriatric patients may arrive with various comorbidities and physiological abnormalities that demand a personalized approach to epidural anesthesia. The aging process leads in many significant changes that influence the administration and efficacy of epidural anesthesia:

Decreased Epidural Space Compliance

1. Fibrosis: The epidural area may become less compliant owing to age-related fibrosis, decreasing the dissemination and efficacy of anesthetics.
2. Calcification: Calcification of ligaments and tissues surrounding the spine may make needle insertion more complex and raise the risk of complications.

Reduced Cardiac Reserve

1. Cardiovascular Changes: Older patients generally have diminished cardiac reserve, increasing the risk of hypotension and other cardiovascular problems during anesthesia.
2. Sensitivity to Vasopressors: Geriatric individuals may be more sensitive to vasopressors and other cardiovascular drugs, demanding cautious titration and monitoring.

Altered Pharmacokinetics

1. Body Composition: Changes in body composition, such as increased fat and reduced muscular mass, alter the distribution and metabolism of anesthetic medications.
2. Renal and Hepatic Function: Declining renal and hepatic function with age effects medication clearance, necessitating modifications in dose and careful monitoring for toxicity.

Drug Dosing and Selection

In geriatric patients, doses of local anesthetics must be carefully controlled to minimize toxicity and extended effects.

Bupivacaine

1. Usage: Bupivacaine is extensively utilized for its lengthy duration of action and acceptable safety profile.
2. Dosing: Lower dosages (0.125% to 0.25%) are frequently adequate to induce effective anesthesia while limiting the risk of toxicity and excessive motor blockage.

Ropivacaine

1. Advantages: Ropivacaine is chosen for its less cardiotoxicity and lower incidence of motor blockage.
2. Dosing: Doses are modified depending on the patient's age, weight, and

renal function, with lower doses (0.2% to 0.3%) generally employed.

Lidocaine

1. Shorter operations: Lidocaine is beneficial for shorter operations because to its fast onset and intermediate duration.
2. Dosing: Lower dosages are utilized to minimize systemic toxicity, with cautious titration depending on the patient's cardiovascular state and general health.

Needle and Catheter Selection

Choosing the proper needle and catheter is critical to avoid trauma and promote effective anesthesia in elderly patients.

Needles

1. Size: Smaller gauge needles (20-22 gauge) are preferable to avoid tissue damage and permit simpler insertion.
2. Approach: The approach should be mild and accurate to minimize harm to the calcified tissues of the elderly spine.

Catheters

1. Flexibility: Flexible, soft-tipped catheters are used to limit the danger of nerve damage and permit easier insertion and placement.
2. Length: Catheter length should be adequate for the patient's size to promote effective anesthetic while limiting the danger of problems.

Monitoring and Safety

Geriatric individuals need close supervision owing to their higher risk of problems.

Vital Signs

1. Continuous Monitoring: Heart rate, blood pressure, and oxygen saturation should be continually monitored to identify any immediate adverse effects.
2. Baselines: Establishing baseline readings pre-procedure assists in recognizing substantial variations post-procedure.

Neurological Assessment

1. Sensory and Motor Function: Regular examination of sensory and motor function is required to achieve the optimal degree of anesthesia and identify any symptoms of neurotoxicity.
2. Cognitive Function: Cognitive function should also be evaluated, since older individuals may be more prone to delirium and other cognitive abnormalities post-anesthesia.

Cardiovascular Monitoring

1. Cardiovascular Status: Close watch for symptoms of hypotension or arrhythmias, with immediate management if indicated.
2. Electrocardiogram (ECG): Continuous ECG monitoring may be necessary for individuals with substantial cardiovascular comorbidities.

Complications and Management

Complications in geriatric individuals might include hypotension, bradycardia, and extended anesthetic effects. Early detection and adequate treatment are critical.

Hypotension

1. Management: Hypotension may be controlled by fluid administration (e.g., crystalloids) and, if required, vasopressors.
2. Monitoring: Close monitoring for indications of fluid excess is required, since older individuals may have impaired cardiac and renal

function.

Bradycardia

1. Intervention: Severe bradycardia may be addressed with atropine, which raises heart rate by blocking the vagus nerve.

Prolonged Anesthesia

1. Monitoring and Supportive Care: Monitoring and supportive care are required until the effects of anesthesia disappear. This involves ensuring the patient is comfortable, warm, and hydrated.

Special Considerations for Frail Elderly Patients

Frail old people constitute a particularly susceptible segment within the geriatric population.

Multimorbidity

1. Comorbid Conditions: Frail elderly individuals generally have many comorbid conditions that might complicate anesthetic treatment.
2. Polypharmacy: Many are on many drugs (polypharmacy) that might interfere with anesthetic agents, demanding careful monitoring and modification of drug regimens.

Nutritional Status

1. Malnutrition: Malnutrition is widespread in the frail elderly and may influence medication metabolism and responsiveness to anesthesia.
2. Preoperative Optimization: Nutritional optimization preoperatively may enhance results and minimize the risk of complications.

Mobility and Functional Status

1. Assessment: Assessing mobility and functional status preoperatively assists in planning postoperative care and rehabilitation.
2. Assistance: Providing proper assistance and resources for postoperative recovery is critical for this vulnerable group.

9.3 Pregnant Patients

Anatomical and Physiological Considerations

Epidural anesthesia is routinely used in obstetric practice for labor analgesia and cesarean births. Pregnant patients provide special difficulties owing to the physiological changes associated with pregnancy.

Increased Epidural Space Pressure

1. Intra-abdominal Pressure: The increased intra-abdominal pressure during pregnancy limits the volume of the epidural space, reducing the distribution and efficacy of anesthetics.
2. Dosing Adjustments: Lower volumes of anesthetic may be necessary to produce the same degree of anesthesia owing to the restricted space.

Enhanced Venous Plexus

1. Vascular Dilatation: Dilated epidural venous plexus raises the danger of inadvertent vascular puncture and systemic absorption of anesthetics.
2. Risk of problems: Increased risk of problems such as high spinal anesthesia or systemic toxicity if inadvertent intravascular injection occurs.

Altered Drug Pharmacokinetics

1. Cardiac Output: Increased cardiac output and blood volume during pregnancy impact the distribution and metabolism of anesthetics.
2. Metabolic alterations: Pregnancy-induced alterations in liver and renal

function may affect the metabolism and excretion of medications.

Drug Dosing and Selection

Choosing the optimum local anesthetic and dosage is crucial in pregnant women to promote adequate analgesia while limiting hazards to both mother and baby.

Bupivacaine

1. Usage: Bupivacaine is extensively used for labor analgesia owing to its lengthy duration of action and dependable safety profile.
2. Dosing: Lower dosages (0.125% to 0.25%) are frequently adequate to induce effective analgesia with reducing motor blockage.

Ropivacaine

1. Advantages: Ropivacaine is recommended for its less motor blockage and lower cardiotoxicity, making it safer for both mother and fetus.
2. Dosing: Doses are modified according on the patient's stage of labor and general health, with lower doses (0.2% to 0.25%) commonly employed.

Lidocaine

1. Cesarean births: Lidocaine is widely used during cesarean births because to its quick onset and intermediate duration.
2. Dosing: Lower doses are recommended to prevent excessive spinal anesthesia and guarantee early beginning of action.

Needle and Catheter Selection

Selecting the suitable needle and catheter is critical to reduce problems and provide adequate anesthesia.

Needles

1. Size: Smaller diameter needles (18-20 gauge) are preferable to avoid tissue damage and the danger of vascular puncture.
2. Approach: The approach should be careful and accurate to minimize injury to the dilated epidural venous plexus.

Catheters

1. Flexibility: Flexible, soft-tipped catheters are used to limit the danger of nerve injury and permit easier insertion and placement.
2. Length: Catheter length should be adequate for the patient's size to promote effective anesthetic while limiting the danger of problems.

Monitoring and Safety

Vigilant monitoring during and after the administration of epidural anesthesia is crucial to guarantee the safety of both mother and fetus.

Vital Signs

1. Continuous Monitoring: Heart rate, blood pressure, and oxygen saturation should be continually monitored to identify any immediate adverse effects.
2. Baselines: Establishing baseline readings pre-procedure assists in recognizing substantial variations post-procedure.

Fetal Monitoring

1. Fetal Heart Rate: Continuous fetal heart rate monitoring is vital to check fetal well-being and identify any symptoms of distress.
2. Response to Anesthesia: Monitoring the fetal response to anesthesia aids in early diagnosis of any detrimental consequences.

Neurological Assessment

1. Sensory and Motor Function: Regular examination of sensory and motor function is required to achieve the optimal degree of anesthesia and identify any symptoms of neurotoxicity.
2. Pain Management: Adequate pain management should be maintained without sacrificing safety for the mother and fetus.

Complications and Management

Complications in pregnant individuals might include hypotension, excessive spinal anesthesia, and fetal discomfort. Prompt identification and treatment are critical.

Hypotension

1. Management: Hypotension may be controlled by fluid boluses (e.g., crystalloids), left lateral position to reduce aortocaval compression, and vasopressors if required.
2. Monitoring: Close monitoring for indicators of fluid excess and fetal distress is required.

High Spinal Anesthesia

1. Intervention: Managed using supportive measures, including head-down posture, supplementary oxygen, and breathing assistance if required.
2. Preventive Measures: Careful titration of anesthetic dosage and periodic aspiration monitoring may help avoid high spinal anesthesia.

Fetal Distress

1. Immediate Intervention: Immediate intervention may involve repositioning the mother, oxygen treatment, and potential emergency delivery if fetal distress is found.
2. Contact: Continuous contact with the obstetric team is vital for prompt

decision-making and action.

Special Considerations for High-Risk Pregnancies

High-risk pregnancies are a particularly vulnerable subpopulation within the obstetric community.

Pre Existing Conditions

1. Comorbidities: High-risk pregnancies may have comorbid illnesses such as hypertension, diabetes, or preeclampsia, which might complicate anesthetic treatment.
2. Medication Interactions: Careful assessment of the patient's medicines and possible interactions with anesthetic drugs is required.

Obstetric Complications

1. Placental Issues: Conditions such as placenta previa or placental abruption may increase the risk of bleeding and need careful monitoring and treatment.
2. Multiple Gestations: Twin or multiple pregnancies may increase the physiological demands on the mother, needing specific anesthetic care.

Intrapartum Monitoring

1. Sophisticated Monitoring: High-risk pregnancies may need sophisticated fetal and maternal monitoring during labor and delivery to guarantee optimum results.
2. Multidisciplinary Approach: Collaboration with obstetricians, neonatologists, and anesthesiologists is vital for handling high-risk pregnancies.

Conclusion

Administering epidural anesthesia in particular populations—pediatric, geriatric, and pregnant patients—requires a full grasp of their unique anatomical, physiological, and pharmacological features. Tailoring medication dose, needle and catheter selection, and attentive monitoring are necessary to guarantee safety and effectiveness. By following best practices and evidence-based standards, physicians may decrease the risk of problems and offer optimum treatment for these vulnerable patient populations. Continuous education, training, and adherence to revised procedures are critical for sustaining high standards of care in the administration of epidural anesthesia in unique populations.

In conclusion, the nuanced knowledge and thorough approach necessary for providing epidural anesthesia to specific groups underline the necessity of specialized training and expertise. Each patient group—pediatric, geriatric, and pregnant—presents distinct problems that necessitate specific tactics to guarantee safety, effectiveness, and best results. By combining extensive patient assessment, accurate medication selection, meticulous technique, and watchful monitoring, healthcare practitioners may traverse these complications and give high-quality, patient-centered care in the area of epidural anesthesia.

Chapter 10

CLINICAL APPLICATIONS OF LUMBAR EPIDURAL ANESTHESIA

Introduction

Lumbar epidural anesthesia is a flexible treatment frequently employed in numerous clinical contexts due to its ability to give adequate pain relief while enabling the patient to stay aware. Its uses span from obstetric anesthetic during labor and delivery, to surgical anesthesia for lower body operations, to chronic pain treatment. This chapter addresses the extensive and thorough clinical applications of lumbar epidural anesthesia, diving into its usefulness in obstetrics, surgery, and pain management, while emphasizing the concepts, procedures, and concerns particular to each application.

10.1 Obstetric Anesthesia Historical Background and Evolution

The use of epidural anesthetic in obstetrics has changed pain management during labor and delivery. Initially developed in the early 20th century, epidural anesthesia has become the gold standard for labor analgesia, offering adequate pain relief while enabling the woman to stay awake and participate fully in the delivery process.

Indications and Benefits

1. Pain Relief During Labor Effective Analgesia: Epidural anesthesia delivers improved pain relief compared to systemic analgesics, enabling the mother to endure a relatively pain-free labor while being completely aware.
2. Mother Satisfaction: High levels of mother satisfaction are connected with the use of epidural anesthesia, leading to a happy delivering experience.

Facilitating Vaginal and Cesarean Deliveries

1. Flexibility: Epidural anesthesia may be modified to give varied degrees of pain relief, from modest analgesia during early labor to total anesthesia for cesarean births.
2. Controlled Analgesia: The capacity to titrate the dose enables for controlled pain management, given the dynamic nature of labor.

Technique and Administration

Pre-procedure Assessment

1. Medical History: A comprehensive medical history, including any contraindications such as bleeding disorders or infections, is important before providing epidural anesthesia.
2. Physical Examination: A focused physical examination, including an evaluation of the lumbar spine, helps detect any anatomical problems that may compromise needle placement.

Patient Positioning

1. Optimal Positioning: Proper positioning of the patient, either in a sitting or lateral decubitus posture, is critical for successful epidural catheter implantation.
2. Comfort and Support: Ensuring the patient is comfortable and

sufficiently supported while placement helps ease the process and lessen anxiety.

Needle Insertion and Catheter Placement

1. Sterile Technique: Maintaining a sterile field is crucial to avoid infections such as epidural abscesses or meningitis.
2. Loss of Resistance method: The loss of resistance method, utilizing saline or air, helps define the epidural space properly.
3. Catheter Advancement: The epidural catheter is gently inserted 3-5 cm into the epidural space, with the location verified by a lack of resistance and negative aspiration for blood or cerebrospinal fluid.

Drug Selection and Dosing
Local Anesthetics

1. Bupivacaine: Commonly used for its extended duration of action and differential block characteristics, providing sensory analgesia with little motor blockade.
2. Ropivacaine: Preferred for its lesser cardiotoxicity and reduced motor blockage, making it acceptable for protracted labor analgesia.

Adjuvant Medications

1. Opioids: Adding opioids such as fentanyl or sufentanil to local anesthetics promotes analgesia and decreases the needed dosage of local anesthetics.
2. Epinephrine: Adding epinephrine may increase the duration of effect and limit systemic absorption of local anesthetics.

Monitoring and Safety

Maternal Monitoring

1. Vital Signs: Continuous monitoring of maternal vital signs, including blood pressure, heart rate, and oxygen saturation, is necessary to identify any harmful effects early.
2. Neurological examination: Regular examination of sensory and motor block levels helps ensure good analgesia and identify any symptoms of problems.

Fetal Monitoring

1. Fetal Heart Rate: Continuous fetal heart rate monitoring is vital to measure fetal well-being and identify any symptoms of distress.
2. Response to Anesthesia: Monitoring the fetal response to anesthesia helps assure the safety of the fetus during childbirth.

Complications and Management

1. Hypotension Prevention and Management: Hypotension is addressed by providing intravenous fluids and, if required, vasopressors such as ephedrine or phenylephrine.
2. Accidental Dural Puncture Management: An accidental dural puncture is handled by conservative methods such as bed rest and fluids, or by conducting an epidural blood patch if a post-dural puncture headache ensues.
3. Respiratory Depression Monitoring and Intervention: Respiratory depression is controlled by lowering the dosage of local anesthetics and giving respiratory support if required.

10.2 Surgical Anesthesia Indications and Benefits
Lower Body Surgeries

1. excellent Analgesia: Epidural anesthesia offers excellent pain management for procedures affecting the lower belly, pelvis, and lower extremities.
2. Reduced Systemic symptoms: Compared to general anesthesia, epidural anesthesia lowers systemic symptoms such as respiratory depression and postoperative nausea and vomiting.

Enhanced Recovery

1. Pain management: Effective pain management with epidural anesthesia may accelerate recovery and minimize the need for systemic opioids postoperatively.
2. Early Mobilization: Patients may mobilize early with epidural anesthesia, minimizing the risk of problems such as deep vein thrombosis.

Technique and Administration

Preoperative Assessment

1. Comprehensive Evaluation: A full preoperative evaluation, including a review of medical history and physical examination, is required to detect any contraindications or possible problems.
2. Informed permission: Obtaining informed permission and discussing the risks, benefits, and alternatives of epidural anesthesia with the patient is vital.

Patient Positioning

1. Optimal posture: Proper posture, either in the lateral decubitus or sitting position, is necessary for effective needle insertion and catheter implantation.
2. Comfort and Support: Ensuring the patient is comfortable and sufficiently supported helps ease the process and lessen anxiety.

Needle Insertion and Catheter Placement

1. Sterile Technique: Maintaining a sterile field is crucial to avoid infections.
2. Loss of Resistance method: The loss of resistance method helps locate the epidural space precisely.
3. Catheter Advancement: The epidural catheter is gently inserted 3-5 cm into the epidural space, with the location verified by a lack of resistance and negative aspiration for blood or cerebrospinal fluid.

Drug Selection and Dosing Local Anesthetics

1. Bupivacaine: Commonly used for its extended duration of action and differential block characteristics, providing sensory analgesia with little motor blockade.
2. Ropivacaine: Preferred for its lesser cardiotoxicity and reduced motor blockage, making it ideal for lengthy surgical operations.

Adjuvant Medications

1. Opioids: Adding opioids such as fentanyl or sufentanil to local anesthetics promotes analgesia and decreases the needed dosage of local anesthetics.
2. Epinephrine: Adding epinephrine may increase the duration of effect and limit systemic absorption of local anesthetics.

Monitoring and Safety
Intraoperative Monitoring

1. Vital Signs: Continuous monitoring of vital signs, particularly blood pressure, heart rate, and oxygen saturation, is necessary to identify any adverse effects early.

2. Neurological examination: Regular examination of sensory and motor block levels helps ensure good anesthesia and identify any symptoms of problems.

Postoperative Monitoring

1. Pain treatment: Continuous evaluation and treatment of pain are necessary to guarantee patient comfort and assist recovery.
2. Complication Detection: Monitoring for any indicators of problems, such as hypotension or respiratory depression, is critical.

Complications and Management

1. Hypotension Prevention and Management: Hypotension is addressed by providing intravenous fluids and, if required, vasopressors such as ephedrine or phenylephrine.
2. High Spinal Anesthesia Management: High spinal anesthesia is handled with supportive measures, including head-down posture, supplementary oxygen, and respiratory assistance if required.
3. Respiratory Depression Monitoring and Intervention: Respiratory depression is controlled by lowering the dosage of local anesthetics and giving respiratory support if required.

10.3 Chronic Pain Management Indications and Benefits
Chronic Pain Conditions

1. excellent Pain reduction: Epidural anesthesia offers excellent pain reduction for chronic pain problems such as chronic back pain, cancer pain, and neuropathic pain.
2. Reduced Opioid Use: By providing excellent pain management, epidural anesthesia may lessen the demand for systemic opioids and their accompanying adverse effects.

Improved Quality of Life

1. Functional Improvement: Effective pain treatment may enhance the patient's functional status and quality of life.
2. Psychological advantages: Pain treatment may also have psychological advantages, lowering anxiety and sadness linked with chronic pain.

Technique and Administration
Patient Assessment

1. Comprehensive Evaluation: A full evaluation, including a review of medical history, physical examination, and pain assessment, is needed to determine the underlying cause of pain and design an effective treatment strategy.
2. Multidisciplinary Approach: Collaboration with other healthcare experts, such as pain specialists, physical therapists, and psychologists, is necessary for complete pain treatment.

Needle Insertion and Catheter Placement

1. Sterile Technique: Maintaining a sterile field is crucial to avoid infections. Loss of Resistance method: The loss of resistance method helps identify the epidural space properly.
2. Catheter Advancement: The epidural catheter is gently inserted 3-5 cm into the epidural space, with the location verified by a lack of resistance and negative aspiration for blood or cerebrospinal fluid.

Drug Selection and Dosing Local Anesthetics

1. Bupivacaine: Commonly used for its extended duration of action and differential block characteristics, providing sensory analgesia with little motor blockade.

2. Ropivacaine: Preferred for its lesser cardiotoxicity and reduced motor blockage, making it ideal for chronic pain treatment.

Adjuvant Medications

1. Opioids: Adding opioids such as fentanyl or sufentanil to local anesthetics promotes analgesia and decreases the needed dosage of local anesthetics.
2. Steroids: Adding steroids may help decrease inflammation and give longer-lasting pain relief.
3. Clonidine: Adding clonidine, an alpha-2 adrenergic agonist, may increase analgesia and give longer-lasting pain relief.

Monitoring and Safety

Pain Assessment

1. Regular Monitoring: Continuous monitoring of pain levels and response to therapy is necessary to guarantee successful pain management and change the treatment plan as required.
2. Patient Feedback: Patient feedback is crucial to assess the success of the therapy and make required modifications.
3. Complication Detection Infection: Monitoring for symptoms of infection, such as fever, redness, or swelling at the catheter site, is necessary.
4. Neurological testing: Regular testing of sensory and motor function helps identify any symptoms of neurotoxicity or other problems.
5. Complications and Management Infection Prevention and Management: Strict adherence to aseptic methods may help avoid infections. If an infection arises, it is handled with medicines and, if required, removal of the catheter.
6. Neurological Complications Monitoring and Intervention: Regular testing of sensory and motor function helps identify any symptoms of neurotoxicity or other problems. Early action, including revision

of the treatment plan or termination of the epidural infusion, may be essential.
7. Systemic Toxicity Monitoring and Management: Systemic toxicity is addressed by lowering the dosage of local anesthetics and providing supportive care as required.

Conclusion

Lumbar epidural anesthesia is a flexible and beneficial method with a broad variety of therapeutic uses. In obstetrics, it offers efficient pain relief during labor and delivery, boosting mother satisfaction and permitting vaginal and cesarean births. In surgery, it gives good anesthetic for lower body operations, decreasing systemic effects and boosting recovery. In chronic pain treatment, it offers efficient pain relief and enhances the quality of life for people with chronic pain problems.

The effective use of lumbar epidural anesthesia needs a full grasp of the concepts, procedures, and concerns relevant to each clinical scenario. By following best practices and evidence-based recommendations, healthcare practitioners may assure the safety and effectiveness of this useful anesthetic approach. Continuous education, training, and adherence to revised guidelines are critical for maintaining high standards of care in the administration of lumbar epidural anesthesia.

Chapter 11

COMPARATIVE TECHNIQUES AND ALTERNATIVES

Introduction

In the area of anesthesia, a number of procedures and options exist, each customized to unique clinical settings and patient demands. Lumbar epidural anesthesia is a cornerstone for many treatments; nevertheless, its efficacy is routinely contrasted with and complimented by other methods such as spinal anesthesia, combined spinal-epidural (CSE) anesthesia, and peripheral nerve blocks. This chapter digs into the complete and extensive comparison of different strategies, covering their principles, administration, uses, benefits, and limitations, offering an in-depth knowledge for doctors to make educated decisions in anesthetic management.

11.1 Spinal Anesthesia Historical Background and Evolution

Spinal anesthesia, also known as subarachnoid block, has a long history extending back to the late 19th century when August Bier first conducted the treatment. Over the years, it has progressed with developments in anesthetic medications, needles, and methods, becoming a frequently used approach for producing deep anesthesia with quick onset.

Indications and Applications

Surgical Procedures

1. Lower Abdominal procedures: Spinal anesthesia is widely used for lower abdominal procedures, including appendectomies and hernia repairs.
2. Pelvic operations: It is particularly useful for pelvic operations such as gynecological procedures and urological surgery.
3. Lower Limb operations: Orthopedic operations affecting the lower limbs, such as knee arthroscopies and hip replacements, benefit from spinal anesthetic.

Obstetric Anesthesia

1. Cesarean Deliveries: Spinal anesthesia is widely used during cesarean sections, giving quick and efficient anesthesia with low danger to the baby.
2. Labor Analgesia: Though less frequent than epidural anesthesia during labor, spinal anesthesia may be utilized for quick start of pain reduction in specific conditions.

Technique and Administration

Pre-procedure Assessment

1. Medical History and Physical Examination: A complete evaluation to uncover contraindications such as infection at the injection site, coagulation problems, or patient refusal.
2. Informed Consent: Discussing the risks, benefits, and alternatives of spinal anesthesia with the patient and receiving informed consent.

Patient Positioning

1. Lateral Decubitus or Sitting Position: Proper placement is vital for effective needle insertion. The sitting posture provides for better

identification of anatomical landmarks, whereas the lateral decubitus position might be more pleasant for the patient.

Needle Insertion

1. Sterile Technique: Maintaining a sterile area to avoid infections.
2. Midline method: The midline method includes putting the needle in the midline of the lower back, generally at the L3-L4 or L4-L5 interspace.
3. Identification of Subarachnoid Space: The needle is advanced until a distinctive "pop" is felt as it goes through the dura mater, and cerebrospinal fluid (CSF) is sucked to confirm placement.

Drug Selection and Dosing Local Anesthetics

1. Bupivacaine: A frequently used long-acting local anesthetic offering efficient sensory and motor block.
2. Lidocaine: A short-acting local anesthetic used for brief treatments.

Adjuvant Medications

1. Opioids: Adding opioids such as fentanyl or morphine to local anesthetics increases analgesia and extends the duration of effect.
2. Vasoconstrictors: Adding vasoconstrictors like epinephrine may extend the effects of local anesthetics by limiting systemic absorption.

Advantages and Disadvantages
Advantages

1. Fast Onset: Spinal anesthesia gives fast onset of anesthesia, generally within minutes.
2. deep blocking: It gives deep sensory and motor blocking, suited for large procedures.
3. Minimal Drug amount: Only a modest amount of anesthetic is

necessary, lowering the danger of systemic toxicity.

Disadvantages

1. Hypotension: A typical side effect related to sympathetic blockage, needing careful monitoring and treatment.
2. Post-dural Puncture Headache (PDPH): A possible consequence, especially in younger individuals.
3. Limited Duration: The duration of anesthesia is limited by the pharmacokinetics of the delivered medications.

11.2 Combined Spinal-Epidural (CSE) Anesthesia Historical Background and Evolution

Combined spinal-epidural (CSE) anesthesia integrates the advantages of spinal and epidural anesthesia, offering quick onset and persistent analgesia. It was initially reported in the 1980s and has subsequently acquired appeal for many surgical and obstetric applications.

Indications and Applications

Surgical Procedures

1. Lower Abdominal and Pelvic procedures: CSE anesthesia is appropriate for procedures needing quick onset and extended anesthesia.
2. Orthopedic Surgeries: It is useful for protracted orthopedic surgeries, giving initial dense blockage with spinal anesthetic and sustained analgesia with epidural infusion.

Obstetric Anesthesia

1. Labor Analgesia: CSE anesthesia is often used for labor analgesia, delivering fast pain reduction with spinal anesthesia followed by continuous epidural infusion.

2. Cesarean Deliveries: It offers good anesthetic for cesarean sections, combining the advantages of quick onset and longer duration.

Technique and Administration
Pre-procedure Assessment

1. Medical History and Physical Examination: A complete examination to detect contraindications and design the anesthetic strategy.
2. Informed Consent: Discussing the dual nature of CSE anesthesia, its advantages, and possible hazards with the patient.

Patient Positioning

1. Optimal Positioning: Positioning the patient in the sitting or lateral decubitus posture to enable needle insertion.

Needle Insertion

1. Sterile Technique: Ensuring a sterile field to avoid infections.
2. Dual Needle procedure: The procedure includes employing a combined spinal-epidural needle set. The epidural needle is put first, followed by the spinal needle via the epidural needle to deliver spinal anesthesia.
3. Catheter insertion: After verifying the spinal needle insertion by CSF aspiration, the epidural catheter is placed into the epidural space for continuous infusion.

Drug Selection and Dosing
Spinal Anesthesia

1. Local Anesthetics: Administering a modest dosage of a local anesthetic like bupivacaine for quick onset of anesthesia.
2. Opioids: Adding opioids to increase analgesia and prolong the duration of effect.

Epidural Anesthesia

1. Continuous Infusion: Using local anesthetics and adjuvants for continuous epidural infusion to sustain extended analgesia.
2. Adjustable Dosing: The epidural catheter enables for dosage modifications depending on the patient's requirements and the operative time.

Advantages and Disadvantages
Advantages

1. Fast Onset and Prolonged Duration: CSE anesthesia delivers the fast onset of spinal anesthesia and the prolonged duration of epidural anesthesia.
2. Flexibility: The ability to titrate the epidural infusion allows flexibility in pain control.
3. Enhanced Analgesia: Combining the approaches promotes analgesia and decreases the needed dosages of local anesthetics and opioids.

Disadvantages

1. Sophisticated Procedure: The procedure is more sophisticated and needs higher expertise and experience.
2. Risk of consequences: Potential consequences include hypotension, PDPH, and infection.
3. Equipment Requirements: The necessity for specific needle sets and equipment might raise prices.

11.3 Peripheral Nerve Blocks

Historical Background and Evolution

Peripheral nerve blocks have a lengthy history, with early procedures documented in the late 19th and early 20th centuries. Advances in anatomical knowledge, imaging technology, and anesthetic drugs have perfected these treatments, making them a standard in contemporary regional anesthesia.

Indications and Applications

Surgical Procedures

1. Upper Extremity procedures: Brachial plexus blocks are widely utilized for shoulder, arm, and hand procedures.
2. Lower Extremity procedures: Femoral, sciatic, and popliteal nerve blocks are employed for knee, ankle, and foot procedures.
3. Trunk procedures: Intercostal and paravertebral blocks are beneficial for thoracic and abdominal procedures.

Pain Management

1. Postoperative Analgesia: Peripheral nerve blocks give good postoperative pain management, lowering the requirement for systemic opioids.
2. Chronic Pain Management: Nerve blocks are utilized for addressing chronic pain problems such as complex regional pain syndrome (CRPS) and neuropathic pain.

Technique and Administration

Pre-procedure Assessment

1. Medical History and Physical Examination: A comprehensive examination to detect contraindications and design the anesthetic strategy.
2. Informed Consent: Discussing the risks, benefits, and alternatives of peripheral nerve blocks with the patient.

Patient Positioning

1. Optimal Positioning: Positioning the patient to expose the target nerve and allow needle insertion.

Needle Insertion and Nerve Localization

1. Sterile Technique: Maintaining a sterile area to avoid infections.
2. Anatomical Landmarks: Using anatomical landmarks and palpation to locate the target nerve.
3. Ultrasound guiding: Ultrasound guiding increases the precision of needle placement and minimizes the risk of complications.
4. Nerve Stimulation: Nerve stimulation may be used to validate needle proximity to the target nerve by eliciting a motor response.

Drug Selection and Dosing
Local Anesthetics

1. Lidocaine: A quick-acting local anesthetic used for diagnostic blocks and brief operations.
2. Bupivacaine and Ropivacaine: Long-acting local anesthetics utilized for extended analgesia and surgical anesthesia.

Adjuvant Medications

1. Opioids with Clonidine: Adding opioids or clonidine may increase analgesia and extend the duration of nerve blocks.

Advantages and Disadvantages
Advantages

1. focused anesthetic: Peripheral nerve blocks give focused anesthetic with little systemic effects.

2. Reduced Opioid Requirements: Effective analgesia minimizes the requirement for systemic opioids and their accompanying adverse effects.
3. Fast Recovery: Patients generally have fast recovery and ambulation compared to general anesthesia.

Disadvantages

1. Technical Complexity: Nerve blocks need expertise and experience for correct needle insertion and adequate anesthetic.
2. Risk of Nerve damage: There is a possible risk of nerve damage, however unlikely with adequate technique and direction.
3. Limited Duration: The duration of anesthesia is limited by the pharmacokinetics of the local anesthetics administered.

Conclusion

The comparative comparison of lumbar epidural anesthesia, spinal anesthesia, combined spinal-epidural (CSE) anesthesia, and peripheral nerve blocks demonstrates a range of alternatives open to anesthesiologists. Each approach has its specific indications, benefits, and limits, making them ideal for diverse therapeutic settings.

Lumbar epidural anesthesia offers flexibility and extended analgesia, making it suitable for labor and postoperative pain control. Spinal anesthetic delivers quick onset and deep block, suited for lower abdominal, pelvic, and lower limb procedures. CSE anesthesia combines the advantages of both approaches, offering quick onset and longer duration, excellent for extensive procedures and labor analgesia. Peripheral nerve blocks give focused anesthetic with little systemic effects, useful for upper and lower extremity procedures and chronic pain treatment.

Understanding the subtleties of these strategies helps practitioners to adjust anesthetic programs to specific patient requirements, maximizing results and boosting patient care. Continuous education, training, and adherence to best practices are critical for maintaining high standards in the delivery of regional anesthetic procedures.

Chapter 12

POSTOPERATIVE CARE AND MONITORING

12.1 Immediate Postoperative Care

After the conclusion of a surgical procedure, the immediate postoperative period is a vital time when diligent monitoring and thorough care are essential to guaranteeing the patient's safety and promoting optimum recovery. This chapter looks into the complete treatment techniques and monitoring procedures adopted during the initial postoperative period, including the spectrum of physiological, psychological, and surgical factors.

Importance of Immediate Postoperative Care

The initial postoperative phase is marked by dramatic physiological changes, including the resolution of anesthesia, the start of pain, and the possible appearance of problems. Effective postoperative care plays a vital role in reducing these problems, enhancing pain management, avoiding complications, and smoothing the transition to recovery. Additionally, thorough surveillance throughout this period permits early diagnosis and action for any adverse events, assuring quick resolution and reducing morbidity and death.

Multidisciplinary Approach

Optimal postoperative care involves a multidisciplinary approach, requiring teamwork among many healthcare specialists, including surgeons, anesthesiologists, nurses, and allied healthcare workers. Each member of the healthcare team offers their skills to meet the different requirements of the patient, guaranteeing complete treatment that spans physical, psychological, and emotional well-being.

Principles of Immediate Postoperative Care

1. Airway, Breathing, and Circulation (ABC): Maintaining airway patency, appropriate breathing, and hemodynamic stability are key elements of early postoperative care. Vigilant monitoring of vital signs, including respiratory rate, oxygen saturation, blood pressure, and heart rate, enables for early diagnosis of respiratory compromise, hypoxemia, or hemodynamic instability. Prompt action, such as airway repositioning, supplementary oxygen supply, fluid resuscitation, or vasopressor support, may be important to stabilize the patient's state and avoid further deterioration.
2. Pain Management: Effective pain management is critical to enhance patient comfort, promote early mobility, and minimize complications such as atelectasis, thromboembolism, and delayed recovery. Multimodal analgesia, including pharmaceutical and non-pharmacological modalities, is widely applied to give synergistic pain relief while avoiding opioid-related adverse effects. Regional anesthetic procedures, such as epidural analgesia, peripheral nerve blocks, or intravenous patient-controlled analgesia (PCA), may be applied to target particular pain pathways and lessen the requirement for systemic opioids.
3. Fluid and Electrolyte Balance: Maintaining fluid and electrolyte balance is critical for sustaining proper tissue perfusion, organ function, and hemodynamic stability. Fluid resuscitation may be necessary to restore intraoperative losses, rectify dehydration, or manage continuing losses from drains or surgical drains. Careful monitoring of fluid intake and output, electrolyte levels, and renal function directs optimum fluid administration and minimizes consequences such as fluid excess, electrolyte imbalances, or renal failure.
4. Surgical Site Care: Optimizing surgical site care is critical to minimize

wound problems, such as infection, dehiscence, or delayed healing. Aseptic methods, including adequate wound dressing and clean handling of surgical tools, limit the risk of infection and enhance wound healing. Regular monitoring of the surgical site for symptoms of infection, inflammation, or hematoma allows for early diagnosis and management to limit consequences.

5. Neurological Monitoring: Neurological monitoring is crucial to examine the patient's neurological health, diagnose any neurological deficiencies, and avoid consequences such as stroke, cerebral ischemia, or nerve damage. Assessment of awareness, orientation, motor function, and sensory perception gives vital insights into the patient's neurological health and informs suitable therapies. Close monitoring for indicators of agitation, disorientation, or localized neurological abnormalities motivates further examination and appropriate management to avoid neurological consequences.

6. Psychological Support: Emotional support and psychological care are key components of early postoperative treatment, addressing the patient's emotional needs, worries, and anxieties. Effective communication, empathy, and reassurance from healthcare practitioners relieve patient discomfort, establish trust, and boost coping strategies throughout the healing process. Psychosocial therapies, such as counseling, relaxation methods, or distraction therapy, may be applied to decrease anxiety, increase mood, and boost general well-being.

7. Nursing Considerations: Nurses play a major role in the administration of early postoperative care, offering watchful monitoring, precise evaluation, and empathetic support to patients along their recovery journey. Nursing issues during the immediate postoperative period include:

8. Vital Signs Monitoring: Regular examination of vital signs, including temperature, pulse, respiration rate, blood pressure, and oxygen saturation, to identify any variations from baseline and prompt appropriate management.

9. Pain Assessment: Comprehensive pain assessment utilizing established

pain scales to determine the severity, location, and characteristics of pain, directing individualized pain management techniques and providing optimum pain treatment.
10. Wound treatment: Diligent examination and treatment of surgical incisions, drainage sites, or wound dressings to avoid infection, improve healing, and permit early diagnosis of wound problems.
11. Fluid & Electrolyte Management: Monitoring fluid intake and output, electrolyte levels, and renal function to maintain proper hydration, electrolyte balance, and renal perfusion, and avoid problems such as fluid excess or electrolyte imbalances.
12. Neurological examination: Regular neurological examination, including level of awareness, orientation, motor strength, sensation, and pupillary response, to identify any neurological deficiencies or changes in neurological state and prompt appropriate management.
13. Psychosocial Support: Providing emotional support, comfort, and advice to patients and their families, addressing worries, fears, or anxieties, and establishing a good coping environment favorable to recovery.

Complications and Interventions

Despite rigorous surgical care, problems may emerge during the initial postoperative period, demanding rapid detection and action to prevent poor outcomes. Common complications include:

1. Respiratory Compromise: Manifested by hypoventilation, hypoxemia, or respiratory distress, respiratory compromise may require interventions such as airway repositioning, supplemental oxygen administration, non-invasive ventilation, or endotracheal intubation to ensure adequate ventilation and oxygenation.
2. Hemodynamic Instability: Characterized by hypotension, tachycardia, or symptoms of insufficient tissue perfusion, hemodynamic instability may demand fluid resuscitation, vasopressor support, or inotropic

medications to restore hemodynamic stability and avoid end-organ damage.
3. Pain Management Challenges: Inadequate pain relief or opioid-related side effects such as respiratory depression, sedation, or nausea may necessitate adjustment of analgesic regimens, including opioid dose titration, adjunctive therapies, or alternative analgesic modalities to optimize pain control while minimizing side effects.
4. Wound Complications: Wound complications such as infection, dehiscence, or hematoma may necessitate wound investigation, debridement, or administration of antimicrobial medication to avoid further deterioration and aid wound healing.

Conclusion
The early postoperative period signals a critical point in the continuity of patient care, when diligent monitoring, detailed evaluation, and fast action merge to ensure patient well-being and nurture optimum recovery. By adhering to the principles of immediate postoperative care and embracing a multidisciplinary approach, healthcare providers can navigate the complexities of the immediate postoperative period with finesse and compassion, ensuring the seamless transition from the operating room to the path of recovery.

12.2 Monitoring and Management of Side Effects

Postoperative care is a key period in patient recovery, needing particular attention to any adverse effects. Ensuring optimum results needs a thorough strategy to monitor and control these side effects, which may profoundly impact the patient's overall experience and health. This section digs into the numerous side effects typically observed post-surgery, offering thorough insights into their monitoring and treatment measures.

Importance of Vigilant Monitoring

The postoperative phase is laden with the potential for severe problems, making watchful monitoring crucial. Timely diagnosis of adverse effects and timely care may avoid progression into more serious difficulties. The objective is to promote patient safety, comfort, and a seamless transition to recovery.

Physiological Side Effects

1. Pain: The Primary Concern: Pain control is a cornerstone of postoperative treatment. Effective pain management is vital not just for patient comfort but also for promoting early mobility and lowering the likelihood of chronic pain development.
2. Monitoring Strategies: Pain Assessment Tools: Utilization of scales like the Visual Analog Scale (VAS) and the Numeric Rating Scale (NRS) for routine pain assessment.

- Patient Feedback: Encouraging patients to share their pain levels and any changes they encounter
- Physical Signs: Observing for non-verbal indicators of pain such as grimacing, restlessness, and changes in vital signs.

Management Approaches:

1. Pharmacological Interventions: Use of multimodal analgesia, mixing opioids, non-opioids (such NSAIDs), and adjuvants (such as anticonvulsants and antidepressants).
2. Regional Anesthesia: Techniques include nerve blocks and epidurals for focused pain relief.
3. Non-Pharmacological Methods: Incorporating physical therapy, cold packs, and relaxation methods.

Nausea and Vomiting: A Common Distress

Postoperative nausea and vomiting (PONV) afflict a considerable proportion of surgical patients, determined by variables such as the kind of

operation, anesthetic medications used, and individual patient sensitivity.
Monitoring Strategies:

1. Regular Assessment: Frequent inquiry regarding nausea and monitoring for indicators of vomiting.
2. Risk Stratification: Identifying high-risk individuals based on criteria like history of motion sickness or past PONV.

Management Approaches:

1. Antiemetics: Prophylactic and therapeutic usage of drugs including ondansetron, metoclopramide, and dexamethasone.
2. Hydration: Ensuring enough fluid balance to avoid dehydration and electrolyte abnormalities.
3. Alternative Therapies: Techniques such as acupuncture and ginger pills.

Hypotension: A Hemodynamic Challenge

Hypotension is a typical postoperative consequence, generally linked to anesthesia, blood loss, or fluid changes. Managing it efficiently is critical to maintain organ perfusion and avoid harmful effects.
Monitoring Strategies:

1. Continuous Monitoring: Using automated blood pressure cuffs or arterial lines for real-time blood pressure surveillance.
2. Volume Status Assessment: Regular examination of fluid status using clinical symptoms and laboratory studies.

Management Approaches:

1. Fluid Resuscitation: Administering intravenous fluids to restore blood volume.

2. Vasopressors: Use of drugs like norepinephrine or ephedrine in situations of prolonged hypotension.
3. Blood Products: Transfusion of blood or blood products if considerable blood loss is discovered.

Respiratory Depression: A Silent Threat

Respiratory depression, sometimes arising from opioid analgesics, presents a considerable danger in the early postoperative period. Ensuring appropriate respiratory function is a fundamental priority.

Monitoring Strategies:

1. Pulse Oximetry: Continuous monitoring of oxygen saturation levels.
2. Capnography: Measuring end-tidal CO_2 for early identification of hypoventilation.
3. Physical Assessment: Regular monitoring of respiratory rate and effort.

Management Approaches:

1. Opioid Sparing Strategies: Utilizing non-opioid analgesics and regional anesthetic to limit opioid usage.
2. Reversal Agents: Administration of naloxone in situations of substantial respiratory depression.
3. Supportive Measures: Oxygen treatment and, if required, non-invasive ventilation or mechanical ventilation.

Psychological Side Effects

1. Anxiety and Distress: Emotional Repercussions
2. Surgical operations and the following recovery may produce substantial anxiety and mental discomfort, affecting overall healing and patient well-being.

Monitoring Strategies:

1. Regular Interaction: Engaging with patients often to measure their emotional condition.
2. Standardized instruments: Utilizing evaluation instruments like the Hospital Anxiety and Depression Scale (HADS).

Management Approaches:

1. Psychological Support: Providing access to counseling services and support groups.
2. Pharmacotherapy: Use of anxiolytics or antidepressants as required.
3. Relaxation Techniques: Encouraging activities such as deep breathing, meditation, and guided visualization.

Depression: A Subtle Burden

Depression may occur as a surgical consequence, especially in individuals with a past history or those facing protracted recovery periods.

Monitoring Strategies:

1. Screening: Routine use of screening measures like the Patient Health Questionnaire (PHQ-9).
2. Patient Communication: Encouraging free talk about emotions and emotional status.

Management Approaches:

1. Psychiatric Consultation: Involvement of mental health specialists for evaluation and therapy.
2. Medication Management: Antidepressant treatment when appropriate.
3. Social Support: Connecting patients with community services and support networks.

Surgical Side Effects

1. Wound Complications: The Healing Challenge
2. Surgical wound complications, including infection, dehiscence, and hematoma, offer substantial difficulties to postoperative rehabilitation.

Monitoring Strategies:

1. Wound Assessment: Regular check for symptoms of infection (redness, swelling, discharge) and healing process.
2. Temperature Monitoring: Checking for fever, which may suggest infection.

Management Approaches:

1. Aseptic Technique: Ensuring rigorous adherence to sterile protocols during dressing changes.
2. Antibiotics: Prophylactic and therapeutic usage of antibiotics depending on culture and sensitivity.
3. Wound Care: Employing sophisticated wound care products and treatments, such as negative pressure wound therapy.

Surgical Site Pain: A Persistent Concern

Surgical site pain, although normal, needs proper care to avoid chronic pain syndromes.

Monitoring Strategies:

1. Pain Diaries: Encouraging patients to keep pain diaries to assess intensity and causes.
2. Regular Evaluations: Frequent examinations by healthcare practitioners to update pain management programs.

Management Approaches:

1. Targeted Analgesia: Local anesthetics and nerve blocks for site-specific pain alleviation.
2. Pharmacological Strategies: Combination of opioids, NSAIDs, and adjuvant medicines.
3. Physical Therapy: Early mobilization and physical therapy to avoid stiffness and enhance recovery.

Conclusion

The rigorous monitoring and control of side effects throughout the postoperative period are crucial in maintaining patient comfort, safety, and best recovery results. A multidisciplinary approach, comprising anesthesiologists, surgeons, nurses, and allied health workers, is vital in addressing the complex interaction of physiological, psychological, and surgical aspects. By applying evidence-based practices and building a patient-centered care environment, healthcare practitioners may successfully negotiate the obstacles of postoperative care, boosting patient satisfaction and supporting successful recovery.

12.3 Long-term Follow-up

While early postoperative treatment is vital, the need for long-term follow-up cannot be emphasized. This phase assures sustained healing, treats any late-onset problems, and supports the patient's return to normality. Long-term follow-up comprises frequent evaluations, continued care of chronic illnesses, rehabilitation, and psychological support.

The Role of Long-term Follow-up

Long-term follow-up is aimed to assess the patient's recovery trajectory, address any residual symptoms, and offer a continuum of care. It strives to detect and resolve issues that may emerge weeks or months following the operation, ensuring that the patient obtains the best possible result.

Chronic Pain Management

Chronic pain may occur as a consequence of surgical intervention, greatly impairing quality of life.

Monitoring Strategies:

1. Regular Assessments: Scheduled follow-up appointments to assess pain levels and response to therapy.
2. Pain Questionnaires: Utilizing instruments like the Brief Pain Inventory (BPI) to quantify pain effect.

Management Approaches:

1. Multimodal Pain Management: Combining pharmacologic and non-pharmacologic therapy.
2. Interventional Procedures: Nerve blocks, spinal cord stimulators, or other pain-relief procedures.
3. Physical treatment: Ongoing physical treatment to enhance function and lessen discomfort.

Rehabilitation and Functional Recovery

Postoperative rehabilitation is crucial in regaining function and fostering independence.

Monitoring Strategies:

1. Functional Assessments: Evaluations by physiotherapists to check improvement.
2. Patient-Reported Outcomes: Tools like the SF-36 to assess quality of life and functional status.

Management Approaches:

1. Tailored Rehabilitation Programs: Customized programs based on

individual requirements and progress.
2. Occupational Therapy: Assisting patients in recovering the capacity to do everyday tasks.
3. Home Exercise Programs: Exercises to continue recovery outside clinical settings.

Psychological Support and Mental Health

The psychological effect of surgery and recuperation may be substantial, demanding continuing mental health treatment.

Monitoring Strategies:

1. Mental Health Screenings: Routine use of instruments like the HADS to detect anxiety and depression.
2. Patient Feedback: Regular talks concerning emotional well-being.

Management Approaches:

1. Therapy Services: Access to psychological therapy or psychiatric treatment.
2. Support Groups: Connecting patients with others who have experienced similar treatments.
3. Medication Management: Antidepressants or anxiolytics as required.

Monitoring for Late Complications

Late problems might emerge far beyond the first surgical phase, demanding attention.

Common Late Complications:

1. Adhesions: Scar tissue that may cause discomfort or blockage.
2. Hernias: Protrusion of an organ through a surgical incision site.
3. Chronic Infection: Persistent or recurring infections at the surgical

site.

Monitoring Strategies:

1. Imaging Studies: CT scans, MRIs, or ultrasounds to discover structural abnormalities.
2. Clinical Assessments: Regular physical exams and lab testing.

Management Approaches:

1. Surgical Interventions: Additional procedures to resolve issues like adhesions or hernias.
2. Antibiotic Therapy: Long-term antibiotics for persistent illnesses.
3. Lifestyle Modifications: Diet, exercise, and other lifestyle adjustments to help healing.

Patient Education and Empowerment

Educating patients on their disease, healing process, and possible problems is crucial for long-term success.

Educational Strategies:

1. Postoperative Care Plans: Detailed plans explaining what to anticipate throughout recovery.
2. Workshops & Seminars: Educational workshops on treating chronic pain, food, and exercise.
3. Resources and Support: Providing access to instructional materials, internet resources, and support networks.

Empowerment Approaches:

1. Encouraging Self-management: Teaching patients how to control their symptoms and spot signals of problems.

2. Shared Decision-making: Involving patients in choices about their treatment to promote adherence and satisfaction.
3. Regular input: Soliciting input to enhance treatment and resolve patient issues swiftly.

Conclusion

Long-term follow-up is a vital component of postoperative treatment, maintaining continued healing and managing any issues that occur. By monitoring chronic pain, supporting rehabilitation, giving psychological support, and educating patients, healthcare practitioners may assist patients achieve the best possible results. This complete approach produces a supportive atmosphere where patients feel empowered and confident in their recovery path, eventually boosting their quality of life.

Chapter 13

ADVANCED TECHNIQUES IN EPIDURAL ANESTHESIA

Introduction

Epidural anesthesia constitutes a cornerstone of contemporary anesthetic treatment, giving considerable pain relief for a number of surgical, obstetric, and chronic pain procedures. As medical technology and practices progress, innovative approaches in epidural anesthesia continue to improve accuracy, safety, and patient outcomes. This chapter goes into three essential areas: ultrasound guidance, fluoroscopy guiding, and continuous epidural analgesia. Each session will address the ideas, procedures, advantages, and clinical applications, delivering a full knowledge for practitioners striving to master these advanced approaches.

13.1. Ultrasound Guidance

13.1.1. Principles of Ultrasound Guidance

Ultrasound guidance has revolutionized regional anesthesia, enabling real-time vision of anatomical features and boosting the accuracy of needle insertion. The theory underlying ultrasonic guiding includes employing high-frequency sound waves to produce precise pictures of tissues, which may be used to guide the insertion of needles and catheters properly.

Understanding Ultrasound Physics

Ultrasound waves are created by a transducer, which transmits and absorbs sound waves. These waves enter the body and are reflected back to the transducer by various tissues, forming a picture depending on the differing densities and acoustic qualities of these tissues. Structures with greater density, such as bone, reflect more sound waves and seem brighter on the ultrasound picture, whereas less dense structures, such as fluid-filled gaps, reflect fewer waves and look darker.

13.1.2. Equipment and Setup

Proper equipment and configuration are critical for efficient ultrasound-guided epidural anesthesia. The important components include:

1. Ultrasound Machine: Modern machines include high-resolution imaging, color Doppler capabilities, and powerful software for image optimization.
2. Transducers: High-frequency linear transducers (5-15 MHz) are often utilized for surface structures, whereas low-frequency curvilinear transducers (2-5 MHz) are employed for deeper structures.
3. Gel: Acoustic gel is applied to the skin to reduce air gaps between the transducer and the skin, boosting picture quality.
4. Sterile coverings: Sterile coverings for the transducer and gel are needed to ensure sterility throughout the process.

The patient is positioned suitably, frequently in a sitting or lateral decubitus posture, to maximize access to the targeted intervertebral area.

13.1.3. Technique of Ultrasound-Guided Epidural Placement

The procedure requires multiple steps:

1. Pre-procedural Planning: The anesthesiologist evaluates the patient's anatomy and identifies the proper intervertebral space.
2. Patient Positioning: The patient is positioned to maximum exposure

of the lumbar or thoracic spine.
3. Probe Placement and Image Acquisition: The transducer is inserted in a transverse or longitudinal configuration across the spine. The spinal processes, laminae, and interlaminar space are recognized. The picture is modified for better viewing of the epidural space.
4. Needle Insertion: Under real-time ultrasound guidance, the needle is moved towards the epidural area. The trajectory is shown, enabling changes to avoid bony structures and guarantee exact implantation.
5. Confirmation of Epidural Space: The loss of resistance method or saline injection is utilized to confirm entrance into the epidural space. Ultrasound may also visualize the distribution of saline or local anesthesia inside the epidural space.

Detailed Steps in Ultrasound-Guided Epidural Placement

1. Pre-procedural Planning: Thoroughly study the patient's medical history and imaging data. Identify any anatomical defects or past surgical modifications that could impact the epidural operation. Select the most acceptable intervertebral space based on clinical reasons and patient anatomy.
2. Patient Positioning: The choice of patient posture (sitting or lateral decubitus) depends on the patient's health and the targeted intervertebral space. Ensure the patient is comfortable and maintain a straight spine to permit good ultrasound imaging.
3. Probe Placement and Image Acquisition: Start with a transverse scan to locate the midline and the spinous processes. Rotate the transducer to acquire a longitudinal picture, positioning the probe with the spinous processes to examine the interlaminar space. Optimize the picture by altering the depth, gain, and frequency parameters on the ultrasound equipment.
4. Needle Insertion: Mark the skin above the specified interlaminar space with a sterile marker. Insert the needle in-plane or out-of-plane,

depending on the practitioner's choice and the quality of the ultrasound picture. Continuously watch the needle tip as it travels towards the epidural area, making real-time changes to avoid bone obstacles.

5. Confirmation of Epidural Space: Use the loss of resistance method with saline or air to confirm penetration into the epidural space. Alternatively, inject a tiny amount of saline under ultrasound guidance to see its distribution inside the epidural area, verifying appropriate needle insertion.

13.1.4. Advantages and Limitations
Advantages

1. Increased Precision: Real-time viewing boosts the precision of needle insertion, lowering the risk of complications.
2. Enhanced Safety: Direct viewing of anatomical features helps minimize vascular and neurological harm.
3. Improved Success Rates: Higher success rates are documented, especially in individuals with difficult anatomy or obesity.
4. Educational Value: Ultrasound guiding gives useful feedback for trainees, aiding the learning process.

Limitations

1. Steep Learning Curve: Mastery of ultrasound-guided procedures needs substantial training and experience.
2. Equipment Cost and Availability: High-quality ultrasound equipment and transducers are costly and may not be accessible in all locations.
3. Operator Dependency: The quality of the ultrasound pictures and the success of the treatment are greatly reliant on the operator's ability and expertise.

13.1.5. Clinical Applications

Ultrasound-guided epidural anesthesia is employed in many clinical scenarios:

1. Obstetric Anesthesia: Ultrasound guidance is extremely effective for labor epidurals, especially in patients with complex anatomy. The ability to view the epidural area and surrounding structures may considerably boost the success rate of epidural catheter insertion in obstetric patients.
2. Thoracic Epidural Analgesia: For thoracic procedures, ultrasonography guidance increases the precision of epidural implantation and boosts postoperative analgesia. Precise catheter placement may lead to improved pain management and perhaps quicker recovery.
3. Chronic Pain therapy: In the therapy of chronic pain problems, ultrasound-guided epidural injections may increase accuracy and effectiveness. This is especially effective for individuals with complicated pain syndromes when correct administration of drugs to the epidural area is critical.
4. Pediatric Anesthesia: In pediatric patients, whose anatomical landmarks are less defined, ultrasonography guidance is crucial for safe and successful epidural anesthesia. The ability to view the epidural space and guarantee correct needle insertion may considerably minimize the risk of problems in this susceptible group.

13.2. Fluoroscopy Guidance

13.2.1. Principles of Fluoroscopy Guidance

Fluoroscopy delivers real-time X-ray imaging, allowing a dynamic image of interior structures during epidural treatments. This imaging approach employs a continuous X-ray beam to generate a succession of pictures presented on a monitor, enabling the practitioner to examine the needle and its relation to bone landmarks and other tissues.

13.2.2. Equipment and Setup

The key components for fluoroscopy-guided epidural anesthesia include:

1. Fluoroscopy Machine: This incorporates an X-ray tube and an image intensifier or flat-panel detector. Modern devices give high-resolution imaging and the capacity to store and retrieve pictures.
2. Radiopaque Markers: These are used to indicate anatomical landmarks on the patient's skin.
3. Lead Aprons and Shields: Protective clothing is important to reduce radiation exposure to the patient and medical personnel.

13.2.3. Technique of Fluoroscopy-Guided Epidural Placement

The procedure involves:

1. Pre-procedural Planning: The target intervertebral space is determined, and radiopaque markers are implanted on the skin.
2. Patient Positioning: The patient is positioned in a manner that maximizes access to the target region, often in a prone or lateral decubitus posture.
3. Fluoroscopy Setup: The fluoroscopy equipment is positioned to offer a good view of the target region.
4. Needle Insertion: Using fluoroscopy, the needle is moved towards the epidural space. Continuous imaging permits real-time changes to avoid bony structures.
5. Contrast Injection: A little quantity of contrast dye is injected to confirm the needle's location inside the epidural space, seeing the distribution of the contrast medium.

Detailed Steps in Fluoroscopy-Guided Epidural Placement

Pre-procedural Planning: Review the patient's imaging data and medical history to identify any anatomical differences or past operations that might affect the surgery. Choose the most acceptable intervertebral space for needle insertion.

1. Patient Positioning: posture the patient prone or in a lateral decubitus posture, assuring comfort and stability. Use cushions or supports to maintain the patient's posture and maximize access to the targeted location.
2. Fluoroscopy Setup: Adjust the fluoroscopy equipment to gain a good image of the spine. Typically, anteroposterior (AP) and lateral views are utilized to advise needle insertion. Confirm the visibility of bone markers and modify the fluoroscopy equipment as appropriate.
3. Needle Insertion: Mark the skin over the target intervertebral region using radiopaque markers. Insert the needle under continuous fluoroscopic guidance, modifying its course to avoid bony structures. Ensure the needle tip approaches the epidural space without entering too deeply.
4. Contrast Injection: Inject a little quantity of contrast dye to confirm the needle's location inside the epidural space. Fluoroscopy will reveal the distribution of the contrast medium, ensuring accurate needle insertion. Adjust the needle as appropriate depending on the contrast pattern.

13.2.4. Advantages and Limitations
Advantages

1. High Precision: Fluoroscopy gives good visibility of bony features, boosting the precision of needle placement.
2. Real-Time Feedback: Continuous imaging enables for fast modifications during needle insertion.
3. Increased Success Rates: Particularly beneficial in individuals with complex anatomy or prior spinal procedures.

Limitations

1. Radiation Exposure: Both the patient and medical personnel are exposed to ionizing radiation, requiring the adoption of protective measures.
2. Cost and Availability: Fluoroscopy equipment is costly and may not be accessible in all clinical settings.
3. Limited Soft Tissue Visualization: Fluoroscopy mainly visualizes bony structures and does not offer comprehensive pictures of soft tissues.

13.2.5. Clinical Applications
Fluoroscopy-guided epidural anesthesia is especially beneficial in:

1. Chronic Pain Management: Fluoroscopy is commonly utilized for epidural steroid injections and other procedures in the management of chronic pain. The capacity to properly distribute drugs to the epidural region might considerably boost pain relief.
2. Spine Surgery: Fluoroscopy is used preoperatively and intraoperatively for spine surgeries. It facilitates the correct positioning of instruments and verification of decompression or fusion methods.
3. Complex Anatomies: Patients with past spinal operations or abnormalities benefit from the precise needle placement given by fluoroscopy. This strategy is particularly beneficial in circumstances when typical landmark-based techniques are hard.

13.3. Continuous Epidural Analgesia

13.3.1. Principles of Continuous Epidural Analgesia
Continuous epidural analgesia includes the implantation of a catheter into the epidural space, allowing for the continuous injection of local anesthetics and/or opioids. This approach gives consistent pain reduction over a long time, making it appropriate for postoperative analgesia, labor pain, and

chronic pain management.

13.3.2. Equipment and Setup
Key components include:

1. Epidural Catheter: A flexible, sterile catheter intended for insertion into the epidural space.
2. Infusion Pump: An electrical device that regulates the pace and amount of medicine administration via the epidural catheter.
3. Sterile Supplies: Including drapes, gloves, and antiseptic solutions to maintain a sterile field during catheter placement.

13.3.3. Technique of Continuous Epidural Analgesia
The procedure involves:

1. Pre-procedural Assessment: Evaluation of the patient's medical history, physical examination, and explanation of risks and advantages.
2. Patient Positioning: The patient is positioned to optimize access to the lumbar or thoracic spine.
3. Catheter Insertion: The epidural space is found using the loss of resistance approach or under ultrasound/fluoroscopy supervision. The catheter is subsequently inserted into the epidural area.
4. Test Dose: A test dose of local anesthetic is provided to check appropriate catheter insertion and to rule out intravascular or intrathecal implantation.
5. Continuous Infusion: The catheter is attached to an infusion pump, and continuous analgesia is commenced. The infusion settings are modified depending on the patient's pain levels and clinical response.

Detailed Steps in Continuous Epidural Analgesia

1. Pre-procedural Assessment: Conduct a comprehensive evaluation of the patient's medical history, concentrating on any contraindications to epidural anesthesia (e.g., coagulation problems, infection at the site of insertion). Discuss the operation with the patient, including possible risks and advantages.
2. Patient Positioning: posture the patient in a sitting or lateral decubitus posture, ensuring the spine is flexed to optimize the intervertebral space. Use supports to maintain the posture and promote patient comfort.
3. Catheter Insertion: Identify the epidural space using the loss of resistance approach with saline or air. Insert the epidural needle at the designated intervertebral location, advance the catheter via the needle, and thread it several centimeters into the epidural space. Secure the catheter in place using adhesive dressings.
4. Test Dose: Administer a test dose of local anesthetic to check appropriate catheter insertion. Observe for indicators of intravascular or intrathecal injection, such as changes in heart rate or blood pressure, and reposition the catheter as appropriate.
5. Continuous Infusion: Connect the catheter to an infusion pump and commence the continuous infusion of local anesthetics and/or opioids. Adjust the infusion settings depending on the patient's pain levels, monitoring for effectiveness and adverse effects.

13.3.4. Advantages and Limitations
Advantages

1. Sustained Pain Relief: Continuous infusion delivers constant and extended analgesia, enhancing patient comfort.
2. Dose Titration: The infusion rate and medication concentration may be changed to fit individual patient demands.
3. Reduced Systemic negative Effects: Localized medication administration lowers systemic absorption and related negative effects.

Limitations

1. Risk of consequences: Potential consequences include catheter migration, infection, and epidural hematoma.
2. Technical Challenges: Proper catheter installation and maintenance need expertise and experience.
3. Patient Monitoring: Continuous monitoring is important to identify and control problems.

13.3.5. Clinical Applications

Continuous epidural analgesia is extensively used in:

1. Postoperative Pain Management: Effective for treating pain following major operations, especially abdominal, thoracic, and lower limb procedures. Continuous epidural analgesia may greatly minimize the requirement for systemic opioids, resulting in fewer adverse effects and a speedier recovery.
2. Labor Analgesia: Provides greater pain relief during labor and delivery compared to systemic analgesics. Continuous epidural analgesia allows for dosage modifications during labor, guaranteeing efficient pain management while protecting mother and fetal safety.
3. Chronic Pain Management: Beneficial for people with chronic pain disorders, allowing for long-term pain management. Continuous epidural infusions may give persistent relief for illnesses such as cancer pain or severe neuropathic pain, enhancing quality of life.

Conclusion

Advanced methods in epidural anesthesia, including ultrasound guiding, fluoroscopy guidance, and continuous epidural analgesia, have considerably advanced the safety, effectiveness, and variety of epidural treatments. Mastery of these approaches involves intensive training, practice, and a complete knowledge of the underlying concepts and clinical applications. As technology continues to progress, these new approaches will surely play an increasingly essential role in current anesthetic practice, enhancing patient outcomes and broadening the boundaries of pain treatment.

Chapter 14

TRAINING AND COMPETENCY IN EPIDURAL ANESTHESIA

Introduction

The practice of epidural anesthesia needs a high degree of competence and knowledge to guarantee patient safety and best results. Achieving expertise in this field demands a solid educational background, intensive training programs, and formal certification and credentialing systems. This chapter presents an in-depth study of these key components, presenting a thorough path for anesthesiologists, trainees, and institutions devoted to excellence in epidural anesthesia.

14.1. Educational Requirements

14.1.1. Foundations of Medical Education

The route to being skilled in epidural anesthesia starts with a thorough medical education. This section highlights the important educational steps, from undergraduate studies to specialist anesthetic training.

Undergraduate Education

A good foundation in the fundamental sciences is necessary for prospective anesthesiologists. Undergraduate education often focuses on:

1. Biology: Understanding the human body at the cellular and systemic levels.

2. Chemistry: Grasping the fundamentals of biochemistry and pharmacology.
3. Physics: Applying ideas of mechanics and waves to understand anesthetic equipment and methods.
4. Mathematics: Developing analytical abilities essential for dose calculations and statistical analysis.

Medical School

Medical school expands on undergraduate studies, offering a complete review of human physiology, pathology, and clinical medicine. Key components include:

1. Preclinical Years: Courses on anatomy, physiology, pharmacology, and pathology give the framework for comprehending the intricacies of anesthesia.
2. Clinical Rotations: Hands-on experience in several medical disciplines, including anesthesiology, gives exposure to patient care and procedural skills.
3. Integrated Learning: Simulation-based training and problem-based learning (PBL) modules increase critical thinking and practical abilities.

14.1.2. Specialized Anesthesia Training

After medical school, specialist training in anesthesiology is needed. This section addresses the essential aspects of residency programs and fellowship possibilities.

Residency Programs

Anesthesiology residency programs offer comprehensive training in all facets of anesthetic practice. Key components include:

1. Clinical Rotations: Rotations in general anesthesia, regional anesthesia, pain management, and critical care.
2. Didactic Education: Lectures, seminars, and case discussions address-

ing the theoretical and practical elements of anesthesia.
3. Simulation Training: High-fidelity simulators for rehearsing complicated operations and handling crises.
4. Mentorship: Guidance and comments from experienced anesthesiologists.

Fellowship Programs

Fellowship programs provide further training in subspecialties, including pain management, pediatric anesthesia, and cardiothoracic anesthesia. These programs often include:

1. Advanced Clinical Training: In-depth exposure to specialty procedures and patient demographics.
2. Research Opportunities: Participation in clinical or fundamental scientific research initiatives.
3. Teaching Experience: Involvement in training residents and medical students.

14.1.3. Continuing Medical Education (CME)

The area of anesthesiology is continually growing, demanding continuing education to keep current with the newest breakthroughs. This section illustrates the relevance of CME.

CME Requirements

1. Licensure Maintenance: Most medical boards need a set amount of CME credits for licensure renewal.
2. Professional Development: CME events, including conferences, seminars, and online courses, give chances for learning and skill building.
3. Certification Maintenance: Board certification in anesthesiology typically includes participation in CME programs as part of the maintenance of certification (MOC) procedure.

Sources of CME

1. Professional Organizations: Organizations like the American Society of Anesthesiologists (ASA) provide a range of CME activities, including yearly meetings, online modules, and journal-based learning.
2. Academic Institutions: Universities and medical institutions conduct CME courses and symposia on the latest research and clinical procedures.
3. Industry Conferences: Medical device and pharmaceutical corporations fund educational programs concentrating on new technology and therapies.

14.2. Training Programs

14.2.1. Structure and Curriculum of Anesthesiology Residency Programs

Residency programs in anesthesiology are meant to give extensive training in all facets of anesthetic treatment. This section explains the structure and content of these programs.

Program Structure

1. Duration: Anesthesiology residency programs normally run four years, including an intern year of general medical training.
2. Rotations: Residents rotate through numerous subspecialties, including general surgery, obstetrics, pediatrics, pain management, and critical care.
3. Progressive Responsibility: As residents move through the program, they acquire increasing degrees of responsibility, culminating in the position of senior resident and team leader.

Curriculum

1. Core Didactics: Weekly lectures and seminars addressing the basics of anesthesia, pharmacology, physiology, and pathology.

2. Simulation Training: Regular sessions utilizing high-fidelity simulators to rehearse procedures and handle complicated clinical settings.
3. Case Conferences: Discussion of tough situations and complications to develop clinical decision-making abilities.
4. Research Training: Opportunities to engage in clinical and fundamental scientific research, including study design, data analysis, and paper writing.

14.2.2. Fellowship Programs and Subspecialty Training

Fellowship programs give advanced training in specialized areas of anesthesiology. This section discusses the numerous fellowship choices and their curriculum.

Types of Fellowships

1. Pain Management: Training in interventional procedures, pharmaceutical therapy, and interdisciplinary approaches to chronic pain.
2. Pediatric anesthetic: Specialized training in the anesthetic treatment of neonates, babies, children, and adolescents.
3. Cardiothoracic Anesthesia: Focused training on anesthesia for heart and thoracic procedures, including enhanced monitoring and perioperative care.
4. Critical Care Medicine: Training in the care of critically sick patients, including enhanced life support, mechanical ventilation, and hemodynamic monitoring.

Fellowship Curriculum

1. Clinical Rotations: Intensive clinical experience in the selected subspecialty, involving hands-on operations and patient care.
2. Didactic Education: Advanced lectures and seminars on specialized issues.
3. Research opportunity: Participation in research initiatives related

to the subspecialty, with opportunity to discuss results at national conferences and publish in peer-reviewed publications.
4. Teaching Responsibilities: Involvement in the instruction and supervision of residents and medical students.

14.2.3. Simulation Training in Anesthesiology

Simulation training is a significant component of current anesthesiology education. This section covers the role of simulation in training programs.

Types of Simulation

1. High-Fidelity Simulators: Mannequins that simulate human physiology and react to medical operations, utilized for rehearsing procedures and handling crises.
2. Task Trainers: Devices meant to imitate certain operations, such as epidural catheter placement or airway monitoring.
3. Virtual Reality (VR) Simulation: Advanced technology enabling immersive experiences for practicing complicated situations and developing procedural abilities.

Benefits of Simulation Training

1. Skill Acquisition: Provides a safe setting for practicing processes and improving technical abilities.
2. Error Management: Allows learners to encounter and handle issues and errors in a controlled context.
3. Team Training: Enhances communication and teamwork abilities via multidisciplinary simulated activities.
4. Evaluation and Feedback: Facilitates objective evaluation of performance and gives chances for focused feedback and improvement.

14.2.4. Mentorship and Professional Development

Mentorship plays a key part in the professional growth of anesthesiologists. This section addresses the significance of mentoring and ways for successful mentorship.

Role of Mentorship

1. Direction and Support: Mentors give direction, support, and encouragement during training and early professional phases.
2. Career Development: Mentors help students career planning, including subspecialty selection, job search, and academic progress.
3. Networking: Mentors assist mentees create professional networks and connect with leaders in the sector.

Strategies for Effective Mentorship

1. Regular Meetings: Establish regular meetings to review accomplishments, objectives, and difficulties.
2. Personalized counsel: Provide individualized counsel based on the mentee's interests, skills, and professional ambitions.
3. Role Modeling: Demonstrate professional demeanor, therapeutic skill, and ethical practice.
4. Comments and Evaluation: Offer constructive comments and assist mentees improve self-assessment and reflection skills.

14.3. Certification and Credentialing

14.3.1. Board Certification in Anesthesiology

Board certification is a marker of professional expertise in anesthesiology. This section covers the certification procedure and its relevance.

Certification Process

1. Written Examination: The first certification test examines knowledge of fundamental and clinical sciences pertinent to anesthesiology.
2. Oral Examination: The oral test examines clinical judgment, decision-

making abilities, and the capacity to handle difficult patients.
3. Clinical Competence: Documentation of successful completion of residency training and evidence of clinical competence.

Significance of Certification

1. Professional Credibility: Certification displays a high degree of skill and dedication to professional standards.
2. Employment Opportunities: Many businesses seek board certification for hiring and privileging.
3. Continued Competence: Certification fosters continued education and skill development via maintenance of certification (MOC) programs.

14.3.2. Maintenance of Certification (MOC)

Maintenance of certification ensures that anesthesiologists keep current with innovations in the profession. This section describes the MOC procedure and requirements.

MOC Process

1. Continuing Medical Education (CME): Participation in CME programs to remain informed with the newest information and practices.
2. Professional Development: Engagement in quality improvement initiatives, peer reviews, and self-assessment.
3. Examinations: Periodic tests to measure knowledge and clinical abilities.

MOC Requirements

1. CME Credits: Completion of a specific number of CME credits throughout each certification cycle.
2. Quality Improvement: Participation in quality improvement activities and documentation of their influence on patient care.

3. Self-Assessment: Regular self-assessment to discover areas for development and drive future learning.

14.3.3. Credentialing and Privileging

Credentialing and privileging protocols guarantee that anesthesiologists are competent to deliver safe and effective treatment. This section addresses these processes and their relevance.

Credentialing Process

1. Verification of Qualifications: Verification of education, training, certification, and license.
2. Professional References: Obtaining references from coworkers and superiors attesting to the anesthesiologist's expertise and professional conduct.
3. Background Checks: Conducting background checks to detect any disciplinary actions or legal difficulties.

Privileging Process

1. Defining Privileges: Determining the exact operations and practices the anesthesiologist is permitted to do.
2. Performance examination: Ongoing examination of clinical performance via peer evaluations, patient outcomes, and incident reports.
3. Reappointment: Regular reappointment and review to guarantee sustained competence and adherence to professional norms.

14.3.4. Institutional Requirements and Standards

Hospitals and healthcare organizations have unique procedures and standards for credentialing and privileging. This section describes these standards and their significance in providing excellent care.

Institutional Policies

1. Credentialing Committees: Institutions often have credentialing committees responsible for assessing applicants and making recommendations.
2. Bylaws and rules: Institutions adopt bylaws and rules describing the credentialing and privileging procedure.
3. Quality Assurance: Institutions establish quality assurance systems to monitor and enhance clinical performance.

Accreditation and Oversight

1. Accrediting Bodies: Organizations such as The Joint Commission (TJC) and the National Committee for Quality Assurance (NCQA) develop criteria for credentialing and privileging.
2. Regulatory Compliance: Institutions must comply with state and federal standards on credentialing and privileging.

14.3.5. Professional Societies and Advocacy

Professional societies play a key role in helping anesthesiologists throughout their careers. This section highlights the role of various societies in lobbying, education, and professional growth.

American Society of Anesthesiologists (ASA)

1. Advocacy: The ASA advocates for policies that promote the profession of anesthesiology and patient safety.
2. Education: The ASA provides a broad variety of educational tools, including CME activities, guidelines, and publications.
3. Professional Development: The ASA offers chances for networking, mentoring, and professional progress.

Other Professional Societies

1. American Board of Anesthesiology (ABA): The ABA controls certifica-

tion and maintenance of certification for anesthesiologists.
2. Specialty Societies: Societies such as the American Society of Regional Anesthesia and Pain Medicine (ASRA) and the Society for Pediatric Anesthesia (SPA) provide specific resources and support.

14.3.6. Global Standards and International Certification

Epidural anesthesia is performed internationally, with varied standards and certification methods. This section discusses global standards and international certification.

International Certification

1. Regional Certification organizations: Many nations have their own certification organizations and protocols for anesthesiologists.
2. International tests: Some anesthesiologists may seek certification via international tests, such as those given by the European Society of Anaesthesiology (ESA).

Global Standards

1. World Federation of Societies of Anaesthesiologists (WFSA): The WFSA supports worldwide standards in anesthesia education, training, and practice.
2. International standards: Development and promotion of international standards and best practices for epidural anesthesia.

Conclusion

Training and expertise in epidural anesthesia are vital to the safe and successful application of this important procedure. Comprehensive educational requirements, organized training programs, and stringent certification and credentialing procedures guarantee that anesthesiologists are well-prepared to offer high-quality treatment. As the industry continues to change, continued education and professional development are vital to sustaining competence in epidural anesthesia.

References

American Society of Anesthesiologists. (2021). Anesthesiology Continuing Education. Retrieved from ASA CME.

European Society of Anaesthesiology. (2020). Certification and Training. Retrieved from ESA Certification.

World Federation of Societies of Anaesthesiologists. (2019). Global Standards in Anesthesia Education. Retrieved from WFSA Standards.

The Joint Commission. (2022). Credentialing and Privileging Standards. Retrieved from TJC Standards.

Neal, J. M., & Hebl, J. R. (2007). Anesthesiology Education and Training. Techniques in Regional Anesthesia and Pain Management, 11(3), 127-133.

Chapter 15

LEGAL AND ETHICAL CONSIDERATIONS IN ANESTHESIA PRACTICE

Introduction

The profession of anesthesia, although tremendously beneficial in improving patient outcomes and enabling difficult medical operations, is intrinsically fraught with legal and ethical issues. These difficulties demand a comprehensive knowledge and attentive application of both legal regulations and ethical principles to assure patient safety, sustain professional standards, and create confidence in the healthcare system. This chapter digs into the complicated terrain of legal and ethical concerns in anesthesia, addressing legal elements, ethical problems, and the crucial significance of precise documentation and record-keeping.

15.1. Legal Aspects of Anesthesia Practice

15.1.1. Regulatory Framework and Professional Standards

Overview of Regulatory Bodies

The practice of anesthesia is controlled by a complicated network of federal, state, and municipal legislation, along with professional standards set out by several accrediting agencies. Key regulatory agencies include:

1. The American Board of Anesthesiology (ABA): Establishes certification

criteria and standards for anesthesiologists.
2. The Joint Commission (TJC): Provides certification and establishes safety and quality requirements for healthcare establishments.
3. State Medical Boards: Regulate medical license and practice within particular states, including the scope of practice for anesthesiologists and nurse anesthetists.

Compliance with Federal and State Laws

Anesthesiologists must handle several federal and state legislation, including:

1. Controlled drugs Act (CSA): Governs the prescription, dispensing, and administration of controlled drugs used in anesthesia.
2. Health Insurance Portability and Accountability Act (HIPAA): Mandates the protection of patient privacy and the confidentiality of medical records.
3. State-Specific Medical Practice Acts: Define the legal scope of practice, licensure requirements, and disciplinary actions for violations.

15.1.2. Informed Consent and Patient Autonomy

Principles of Informed Consent

Informed consent is a fundamental legal and ethical requirement in anesthesia practice. It involves:

1. Disclosure: Providing comprehensive information about the anesthesia procedure, including risks, benefits, and alternatives.
2. Comprehension: Ensuring that the patient understands the information provided.
3. Voluntariness: Securing the patient's voluntary agreement to proceed without coercion.

Legal Implications of Informed Consent

Failure to obtain proper informed consent can lead to legal repercussions, including:

1. Malpractice Claims: Patients may file lawsuits for alleged negligence if they suffer harm without being adequately informed of the risks.
2. Disciplinary Actions: Regulatory bodies may impose sanctions or revoke licensure for breaches in obtaining informed consent.

15.1.3. Malpractice and Liability

Elements of a Malpractice Claim
To establish a malpractice claim, the following elements must be proven:

1. Duty of Care: The anesthesiologist owed a duty of care to the patient.
2. Breach of Duty: The anesthesiologist breached the standard of care.
3. Causation: The breach directly caused the patient's injury.
4. Damages: The patient suffered actual harm or damages as a result.

Risk Management Strategies

To mitigate the risk of malpractice claims, anesthesiologists should:

1. Adhere to Standards of Care: Follow established norms and practices.
2. Engage in Continuing Education: Stay updated with the latest advancements and best practices.
3. Maintain Clear Communication: Ensure thorough and open communication with patients and healthcare team members.
4. Document Thoroughly: Keep accurate and complete records of all patient contacts and procedures.

15.1.4. Legal Responsibilities in Emergency Situations

Good Samaritan Laws
Good Samaritan laws give legal protection to healthcare practitioners

who provide emergency treatment in good faith. Key elements include:

1. Scope of Protection: These regulations often cover activities done during crises outside the provider's customary therapeutic context.
2. Limitations: Protection is typically restricted to treatment delivered without severe negligence or reckless behavior.

Obligations in the Operating Room

In emergency scenarios inside the operating room, anesthesiologists have a legal responsibility to:

1. Act Promptly: Respond immediately to emergency situations to stabilize the patient.
2. Follow Protocols: Adhere to established emergency procedures and standards.
3. Document Actions: Record all actions done and their reasoning in the patient's medical record.

15.2. Ethical Issues

15.2.1. Principles of Biomedical Ethics

Autonomy

Respecting patient autonomy involves:

1. Informed Consent: Ensuring patients are fully informed and consenting willingly.
2. Shared Decision-Making: Engaging patients in choices about their treatment, respecting their beliefs and preferences.

Beneficence

The concept of beneficence demands anesthesiologists to:

1. Promote Well-Being: Act in the best interest of the patient to maximize

benefits and minimize risks.
2. Evidence-Based Practice: Use the best available evidence to inform healthcare choices.

Non-Maleficence

Non-maleficence, or "do no harm," dictates that anesthesiologists:

1. Avoid Unnecessary Risks: Take precautions to avoid possible risks connected with anesthesia.
2. Continuous Monitoring: Vigilantly monitor patients to rapidly detect and handle adverse occurrences.

Justice

Justice in anesthesiology practice involves:

1. Equitable treatment: Providing fair and equitable treatment regardless of a patient's history or socioeconomic situation.
2. Resource Allocation: Making fair judgments on the allocation of scarce resources, such as critical care beds or specialized therapies.

15.2.2. Confidentiality and Patient Privacy

HIPAA and Confidentiality

Maintaining patient anonymity is both a legal necessity under HIPAA and an ethical commitment. Key factors include:

1. Data Security: Implementing procedures to secure patient information from unauthorized access or breaches.
2. Information Sharing: Disclosing patient information only with permission or when legally required.

Ethical Challenges in Confidentiality

Anesthesiologists may confront ethical difficulties relating to secrecy, such as:

1. Disclosure to Family Members: Balancing the necessity for family interaction with the patient's right to privacy.
2. Reporting Obligations: Navigating obligatory reporting obligations for specific situations (e.g., communicable diseases) while protecting patient confidentiality.

15.2.3. End-of-Life Decisions and Palliative Care Advance Directives and Do-Not-Resuscitate (DNR) Orders

Respecting patient autonomy in end-of-life care involves:

1. Advance Directives: Adhering to patients' desires as indicated in advance directives governing the use of life-sustaining therapies.
2. DNR Orders: Honoring DNR instructions and ensuring all team members are aware of and obey these directions throughout surgical and anesthetic treatment.

Palliative Care and Ethical Considerations

Anesthesiologists play a key role in palliative care by:

1. Pain Management: Providing efficient pain treatment and symptom management for terminally ill patients.
2. Ethical Decision-Making: Navigating challenging ethical considerations involving the balance between reducing pain and perhaps hastening death.

15.2.4. Ethical Dilemmas in Clinical Practice Informed Refusal Patients have the right to reject treatment, and anesthesiologists must:

1. Respect Decisions: Honor the patient's informed refusal, even if it

contrasts with medical advice.
2. Provide Alternatives: Offer alternate choices and ensure the patient knows the possible ramifications of rejection.

Dual Loyalties

Anesthesiologists may confront conflicts of interest between:

1. Patient Advocacy: Prioritizing the patient's best interests.
2. Institutional Obligations: Balancing duties to the healthcare institution, such as resource distribution or cost control.

15.3. Documentation and Record-Keeping

15.3.1. Importance of Accurate Documentation
Legal and Ethical Imperatives
Accurate documentation is vital for:

1. Legal Protection: Providing proof of adherence to standards of care and informed consent.
2. Ethical responsibility: Ensuring openness and responsibility in patient care.

Enhancing Patient Safety

Thorough documentation promotes patient safety by:

1. Communication: Facilitating clear communication among healthcare team members.
2. Continuity of Care: Ensuring complete and continuous care across diverse providers and locations.

15.3.2. Components of Effective Documentation
Preoperative Documentation

Key factors include:

1. Patient Assessment: Detailed history and physical examination results.
2. Informed Consent: Documentation of the informed consent process, including discussions of risks, benefits, and alternatives.
3. Anesthesia Plan: The planned anesthesia approach, including medications, techniques, and anticipated challenges.

Intraoperative Documentation

Essential components involve:

1. Vital Signs and Monitoring: Continuous recording of vital signs, anesthetic agents administered, and monitoring data.
2. Procedural Details: Detailed account of procedures performed, including any deviations from the planned approach and rationale.
3. Adverse Events: Documentation of any intraoperative complications and the actions taken to address them.

Postoperative Documentation

Critical aspects include:

1. Recovery Status: Patient's condition and vital signs in the immediate postoperative period.
2. Pain Management: Documentation of pain levels, analgesic administration, and response to treatment.
3. Complications and Follow-Up: Any postoperative complications and the plans for follow-up care.

15.3.3. Electronic Health Records (EHRs)

Advantages of EHRs EHRs offer numerous benefits, such as:

1. Accessibility: Immediate access to patient records by all authorized

healthcare professionals.
2. Integration: Integration of data from diverse sources, offering a full perspective of the patient's medical history.
3. Error Reduction: Reduction in documentation mistakes and enhanced readability compared to paper records.

Challenges and Considerations
Despite their benefits, EHRs face obstacles, including:

1. User Interface Issues: Complex interfaces may limit effective documentation and workflow.
2. Data Security: Ensuring patient data privacy and protection against cybersecurity risks.
3. Training Needs: Adequate training for healthcare practitioners to utilize EHR systems successfully and reduce mistakes.

15.3.4. Legal Standards for Documentation Legibility and Accuracy
Documentation must be:

1. Legible: Easily readable to guarantee clarity and understanding.
2. Accurate: Reflective of the patient's condition, treatment delivered, and reaction to interventions.

Timeliness and Completeness
Documentation should be:

1. Timely: Entered soon following patient contacts to ensure accuracy and relevance.
2. Complete: Include all important information required for continuity of care and legal responsibility.

Authentication and Signatures

Entries in patient records should be:

1. Authenticated: Clearly credited to the relevant healthcare practitioner.
2. Signed and Dated: With electronic signatures or handwritten signatures and dates as relevant.

15.3.5. Risk Management Strategies

Standardization of Documentation Practices
Standardizing documentation:

1. Templates and Checklists: Use standardized templates and checklists to guarantee consistency and thoroughness.
2. Quality Assurance Measures: Implement frequent audits and reviews of documentation procedures to identify opportunities for improvement.

Communication and Interdisciplinary Collaboration

Effective communication:

1. Interdisciplinary Communication: Facilitate communication among members of the healthcare team to enable coordinated treatment and proper documentation.
2. Patient Engagement: Involve patients in their treatment and urge them to engage in the documentation process, such as by evaluating their records for correctness.

Ongoing Training and Education

Continued education:

1. Training Programs: Offer continuing training and instruction for healthcare practitioners on documenting best practices, EHR systems, and legal requirements.

2. Feedback Mechanisms: Establish systems for feedback and peer review to support continual improvement in documentation quality.

Conclusion

Legal and ethical issues are present in every phase of anesthetic practice, from gaining informed permission to recording patient treatment. Anesthesiologists must traverse complicated regulatory frameworks, enforce ethical values, and keep thorough documentation to guarantee patient safety, limit legal risks, and sustain professional standards. By accepting these obligations with dedication and honesty, anesthesiologists contribute to the delivery of high-quality treatment and the maintenance of patient confidence in the healthcare system.

Chapter 16

RESEARCH AND FUTURE DIRECTIONS

16.1: Current Research Trends

In the persistent quest of better patient outcomes and refining clinical methods, the discipline of epidural anesthesia sits at the forefront of medical research. This section digs into the current research trends impacting the landscape of epidural anesthesia, investigating the newest developments, creative approaches, and potential paths of investigation.

16.1.1: Pharmacological Innovations

Expanding Horizons of Analgesic Agents

The hunt for safer, more effective analgesic medications continues to drive pharmacological research in epidural anesthesia. Within this domain, innovative chemicals and formulations are under evaluation for their potential to change pain treatment practices. Among them, alpha-2 agonists such as dexmedetomidine and clonidine have received great attention for their potential to extend analgesia and minimize opioid intake when administered as adjuvants to local anesthetics. Their unique method of action, which includes regulation of central pain pathways, shows promise for alleviating both acute and chronic pain states.

Similarly, the research of neuromodulators, including N-methyl-D-aspartate (NMDA) receptor antagonists and gabapentinoids, indicates a paradigm shift towards focused pain treatment techniques. By selectively targeting certain pain pathways, these medicines provide the opportunity for personalized analgesic regimes that reduce unwanted effects and enhance patient outcomes. Ongoing research initiatives attempt to identify the appropriate dose, timing, and combination treatments using various pharmacological substances, with the ultimate objective of enhancing pain relief while minimizing side effects and consequences.

Advancements in Liposomal Formulations

Liposomal formulations provide a cutting-edge strategy to drug administration, giving the benefits of sustained release and longer duration of action. In the field of epidural anesthesia, liposomal formulations of local anesthetics have emerged as a viable path for increasing the duration of pain relief while avoiding systemic toxicity. By encapsulating local anesthetics inside lipid bilayers, liposomal formulations permit controlled release of the medication over a protracted time, so extending the duration of analgesia and eliminating the need for frequent dosage.

Current research efforts in this sector are focused on improving liposomal delivery methods to enhance effectiveness and safety. Key areas of investigation include optimizing the lipid content, particle size, and surface features of liposomes to optimize medication encapsulation and release kinetics. Additionally, efforts into innovative liposomal formulations that combine adjuvants or synergistic compounds seek to further increase the analgesic benefits while limiting systemic exposure and toxicity. As these research attempts develop, liposomal formulations have the potential to alter the landscape of epidural anesthesia, enabling persistent pain relief and better patient outcomes across a variety of clinical situations.

16.1.2: Advancements in Regional Anesthesia Techniques
  Precision via Ultrasound Guidance

The development of ultrasound-guided regional anesthetic procedures has revolutionized the landscape of pain treatment, giving remarkable precision and accuracy in nerve location and blockage. By giving real-time vision of anatomical structures and needle trajectory, ultrasound guidance helps doctors to accurately target nerve plexuses and decrease the danger of unintentional damage or arterial puncture. This greater accuracy not only enhances the efficiency of nerve blocks but also minimizes the occurrence of complications such as nerve injury and hematoma development.

Current research activities in this area are focused on perfecting ultrasound-guided procedures for a variety of nerve blocks, including upper and lower extremity blocks, truncal blocks, and neuraxial blocks. Investigations exploring innovative ways for maximizing needle visualization, strengthening nerve identification algorithms, and combining modern imaging modalities show promise for further boosting the accuracy and effectiveness of ultrasound-guided regional anesthetic. Additionally, research initiatives are ongoing to study the relevance of ultrasound-guided procedures in unique patient groups, such as pediatric and obstetric patients, where standard landmark-based approaches may be problematic or less dependable.

Harnessing the Potential of Continuous Catheter Infusion

Continuous infusion methods, enabled by indwelling catheters, provide a way of giving sustained analgesia for postoperative pain control. By continually providing local anesthetics or analgesic drugs directly to the site of nerve blockage, continuous catheter infusion methods offer persistent pain relief while avoiding the need for frequent bolus dosage. This not only increases patient comfort and satisfaction but also minimizes the danger of systemic toxicity associated with high-dose opioid analgesia.

Current research efforts in this sector are focused on refining catheter insertion procedures, infusion rates, and pharmaceutical combinations to enhance effectiveness while reducing problems such as catheter dislodgement and infection. Additionally, efforts into innovative catheter designs, such multiorifice catheters and drug-eluting catheters, seek to increase drug distribution and extend the duration of analgesia. By exploiting the potential of continuous catheter infusion methods, researchers strive to increase the quality of postoperative pain management and boost patient outcomes after surgery.

16.1.3: Innovations in Enhanced Recovery After Surgery (ERAS)

Multimodal Analgesia Strategies

Multimodal analgesia, which includes the use of various analgesic medications with varied mechanisms of action, sits at the core of improved recovery after surgery (ERAS) protocols. By addressing several pain pathways concurrently, multimodal analgesia regimens give greater pain relief while limiting the negative effects associated with individual drugs. Current research trends in this field concentrate on improving the selection and combination of analgesic drugs to enhance effectiveness and reduce unwanted effects.

In particular, investigations into novel combinations of pharmacological agents, including nonsteroidal anti-inflammatory drugs (NSAIDs), acetaminophen, and gabapentinoids, aim to achieve synergistic effects that enhance pain relief without increasing the risk of complications such as gastrointestinal bleeding or renal impairment. Additionally, research efforts are ongoing to study the function of adjuvant treatments, including as regional anesthetic procedures and intravenous lidocaine infusions, in boosting the analgesic benefits of multimodal regimens. By developing multimodal analgesia techniques, researchers hope to maximize postoperative pain management and allow early recovery after surgery.

Integration of Enhanced Monitoring Technologies

Advancements in monitoring technology provide new options for improving perioperative treatment and boosting patient outcomes within the framework of ERAS procedures. By offering real-time monitoring of patients' physiological indicators and pain levels, these technologies help doctors to detect and resolve difficulties rapidly, therefore lowering the risk of adverse events and encouraging early recovery.

Current research efforts in this area concentrate on integrating wearable devices, remote monitoring systems, and telemedicine platforms into

ERAS pathways to promote continuous monitoring and early intervention. Wearable devices integrated with biosensors give the capacity to assess vital signs, activity levels, and pain ratings in real time, offering crucial insights into patients' postoperative recovery trajectories. Similarly, remote monitoring systems allow for the smooth transfer of data from patients' homes to healthcare practitioners, allowing prompt revisions to treatment plans and interventions as required.

Conclusion

In conclusion, the area of epidural anesthesia continues to grow at a fast rate, driven by continuous research initiatives, technology breakthroughs, and creative clinical procedures. Current research trends in pharmaceutical advances, regional anesthetic methods, and better recovery tactics show promise for altering the landscape of pain treatment and increasing patient outcomes across a variety of clinical settings. By embracing these trends and supporting multidisciplinary cooperation, researchers and clinicians alike may strive towards the common aim of maximizing pain treatment, boosting patient happiness, and aiding early recovery after surgery.

16.2: Innovations in Epidural Anesthesia

Innovation is the pulse of development in medicine, moving the field of epidural anesthesia into unparalleled realms of effectiveness, safety, and patient-centered care. This section begins on a trip into the domain of innovation, investigating the newest breakthroughs, innovative approaches, and imaginative ambitions redefining the landscape of epidural anesthesia.

16.2.1: Precision Through Targeted Drug Delivery Systems

Epidural Drug Delivery Pumps: Unlocking Precision and Control

Implantable drug delivery pumps signal a new age of precision in epidural anesthesia, allowing practitioners unrivaled control over medicine administration directly to the spinal area. These complex gadgets, comparable to microscopic reservoirs of medicinal potential, are a triumph of biomedical engineering and pharmacological elegance.

The premise underpinning epidural drug delivery pumps is deceptively simple: deliver the appropriate medicine, in the right amount, to the right spot, at the right time. By implanting these devices into the epidural space, doctors may obtain targeted and prolonged release of analgesic drugs, bypassing the systemic circulation and lowering the danger of systemic adverse effects.

Current research initiatives in this sector are complex, covering breakthroughs in pump design, medication formulations, and programmable infusion algorithms. Efforts are ongoing to build smarter pumps capable of reacting to patients' shifting pain trajectories, modifying infusion rates in real-time depending on physiological indicators and patient-reported results. Through the convergence of technical creativity and pharmaceutical innovation, epidural medication delivery pumps have the potential to transform pain treatment, providing patients a road to continuous relief and enhanced quality of life.

Closed-Loop Systems: Melding Technology with Therapeutics

Closed-loop systems represent the ultimate synergy between technology and medicine, leveraging the power of real-time feedback mechanisms to improve medication administration and increase patient outcomes. At the core of these systems lies a complex dance between sensors, algorithms, and actuators, coordinated with precision to give individualized care suited to each patient's specific requirements.

In the field of epidural anesthesia, closed-loop devices provide a tantalizing view into the future of pain treatment, promising to transform the way analgesic drugs are delivered and titrated. By continually monitoring patients' physiological reactions and pain levels, these systems may dynamically change drug delivery settings, fine-tuning infusion rates and dosing regimens to produce optimum analgesia while reducing the risk of adverse effects and overdose.

Current research efforts in closed-loop epidural anesthetic systems are focused on developing computational algorithms and sensor technology to better accuracy and dependability. Advanced machine learning algorithms, trained on enormous repositories of patient data, offer the potential to find subtle patterns and connections, allowing predictive modeling of pain trajectories and preventative therapies. As these systems expand and mature, they offer the possibility of changing the practice of epidural anesthesia, ushering in an era of individualized pain management adapted to each patient's specific physiology and preferences.

16.2.2: Harnessing the Power of Neurostimulation Techniques

Epidural Electrical Stimulation: Illuminating Pathways to Pain Relief

Epidural electrical stimulation stands as a light of hope in the domain of chronic pain treatment, delivering a lifeline to patients suffering with intractable pain problems. At its foundation, epidural electrical stimulation includes the administration of low-voltage electrical impulses to specified portions of the spinal cord, regulating pain signals and restoring balance to aberrant neural circuits.

The therapeutic potential of epidural electrical stimulation encompasses a wide range of chronic pain syndromes, including neuropathic pain, failed back surgery syndrome, and complex regional pain syndrome (CRPS). By engaging with the spinal cord's complicated network of neurons, these electrical impulses may interrupt maladaptive pain pathways, allowing sufferers reprieve from the continuous grip of chronic pain.

Current research attempts in epidural electrical stimulation are focused on optimizing stimulation settings, electrode designs, and targeting tactics to enhance effectiveness and reduce adverse effects. Innovations such as high-definition electrode arrays and adaptive stimulation algorithms offer the potential of boosting spatial specificity and temporal accuracy, allowing doctors to precisely target pain circuits while preserving surrounding brain structures.

Peripheral Nerve Stimulation: Navigating the Frontiers of Pain Relief

Peripheral nerve stimulation is a diverse modality in the armamentarium of pain therapy, enabling targeted relief for a plethora of pain syndromes emerging from peripheral nerve dysfunction. Unlike epidural electrical stimulation, which targets pain signals at the level of the spinal cord, peripheral nerve stimulation sends electrical impulses directly to peripheral nerves, intercepting pain signals before they reach the central nervous system.

The therapeutic uses of peripheral nerve stimulation are wide-ranging, embracing disorders such as postoperative pain, neuropathic pain, and CRPS. By carefully altering the activity of peripheral nerves, these electrical impulses may interrupt faulty pain signaling pathways, affording patients a relief from the unrelenting cycle of pain and misery.

Current research efforts in peripheral nerve stimulation are complex, including electrode design, stimulation settings, and targeting techniques. Novel electrode topologies, such as paddle leads and 3D-printed arrays, offer the potential to increase spatial specificity and selectivity, allowing doctors to precisely target particular neurons while reducing off-target effects. Additionally, developments in stimulation algorithms, including burst and high-frequency stimulation, seek to enhance pain treatment while reducing power consumption and battery depletion.

16.2.3: Exploring the Frontiers of Nanotechnology and Biomaterials

Nanoparticle-Based Drug Delivery: Miniaturizing Therapeutic Potential

Nanoparticle-based drug delivery systems represent a paradigm change in the area of drug delivery, giving a pathway to precision medicine and individualized therapies. At their heart, nanoparticles are minuscule carriers capable of encapsulating therapeutic chemicals and delivering them to particular anatomical areas with unparalleled accuracy and efficiency.

In the context of epidural anesthesia, nanoparticle-based drug delivery methods have tremendous potential for increasing the effectiveness and safety of analgesic drugs. By encapsulating analgesic medications into biocompatible nanoparticles, researchers may achieve prolonged release and tailored distribution to the epidural area, reducing systemic exposure and boosting therapeutic effectiveness.

Current research efforts in nanoparticle-based drug delivery are focused on refining nanoparticle design, surface modification, and drug loading techniques to increase drug encapsulation and release kinetics. Advanced nanomaterials, such as liposomes, polymeric nanoparticles, and lipid-based carriers, provide diverse platforms for modifying drug delivery features to particular therapeutic demands. Through careful control of particle size, surface charge, and drug release kinetics, researchers may fine-tune nanoparticle compositions to achieve optimum therapeutic results while avoiding off-target effects and systemic toxicity.

Biomaterial Implants: Building Bridges to Tissue Regeneration

Biomaterial implants provide a novel method to tissue engineering and regenerative medicine, enabling new pathways for healing and replacing damaged tissues inside the epidural region. These unique constructions, constructed from biocompatible materials such as polymers, hydrogels, and scaffolds, serve as platforms for targeted medication delivery, cell transplantation, and tissue regeneration.

In the field of epidural anesthesia, biomaterial implants show promise for addressing a variety of clinical difficulties, from postoperative pain control to spinal cord damage repair. By incorporating medicinal drugs, growth factors, and stem cells into biomaterial scaffolds, researchers may construct multifunctional implants capable of encouraging tissue repair, controlling inflammation, and supporting neuronal regeneration.

Current research efforts in biomaterial implants are focused on improving implant design, material composition, and biodegradation kinetics to increase biocompatibility and tissue integration. Advanced manufacturing methods, including 3D printing and electrospinning, give fine control over implant design and porosity, enabling researchers to adapt mechanical characteristics and drug release patterns to particular clinical applications.

Conclusion: Charting the Course for Future Innovation

Innovation is the lifeblood of advancement in epidural anesthesia, moving the discipline towards new frontiers of effectiveness, safety, and patient-centered care. From precise medication delivery systems to sophisticated neurostimulation methods and biomaterial implants, the future of epidural anesthesia is loaded with promise and possibility.

As researchers continue to push the bounds of knowledge and explore the frontiers of science, it is vital to maintain a strong commitment to ethical practice, patient safety, and multidisciplinary cooperation. By embracing innovation, promoting creativity, and supporting a culture of continuous learning, the profession of epidural anesthesia may continue to expand and thrive, bringing transforming solutions to patients in need.

In this age of tremendous scientific discovery and technological growth, the possibilities are boundless. By leveraging the power of innovation, we can design a future where pain is treated with accuracy, compassion, and humanity, helping patients to live richer, healthier lives.

16.3: Future Prospects

In the ever-evolving environment of medicine, the future is a canvas of unlimited possibilities, where innovation and discovery collide to create the direction of healthcare. This section goes on a voyage into the world of future possibilities in epidural anesthesia, covering new trends, innovative notions, and transformational technology set to change the practice of pain management and perioperative care.

16.3.1: Precision Medicine: Charting New Frontiers

Pharmacogenomics: Personalizing Pain Management

Pharmacogenomics has the possibility of transforming pain management by personalizing therapy regimens to individual genetic profiles. By deciphering the complicated interaction between genetic differences and pharmacological responses, researchers may find genetic markers predictive of individual reactions to analgesic drugs, allowing tailored treatment regimens that enhance effectiveness and reduce unwanted effects.

The incorporation of pharmacogenomic data into clinical practice has the potential to alter the area of epidural anesthesia, affording doctors significant insights into individuals' genetic predispositions and drug metabolic pathways. Armed with this information, practitioners may make educated choices about medication selection, dose, and titration, ensuring that each patient gets the most effective and well-tolerated analgesic regimen.

Predictive Modeling: Anticipating Pain Trajectories

Predictive modeling approaches, backed by artificial intelligence and machine learning algorithms, give a look into the future of pain treatment. By examining huge repositories of patient data, including demographics, clinical factors, and treatment results, predictive algorithms may project patients' pain trajectories and identify those at risk of poor outcomes.

In the field of epidural anesthesia, predictive modeling offers the potential to improve perioperative pain control measures and better patient outcomes. By employing predictive algorithms to forecast pain severity, duration, and response to therapy, doctors may proactively intervene to alleviate pain and enhance recovery trajectories. Through the incorporation of predictive modeling into clinical decision-making processes, epidural anesthesia may grow into a genuinely patient-centric discipline, suited to each individual's specific requirements and preferences.

16.3.2: Regenerative Medicine: Healing from Within

Stem Cell Therapy: Unlocking the Power of Regeneration

Stem cell therapy provides a paradigm change in the treatment of spinal cord injuries and chronic pain syndromes, having the possibility to restore function and reduce symptoms via tissue regeneration. By exploiting the regenerative power of stem cells, researchers seek to heal damaged neural tissue, boost axonal regeneration, and restore sensory and motor function in patients with spinal cord injuries.

In the field of epidural anesthesia, stem cell treatment has potential for boosting the efficiency of pain control therapies and aiding tissue healing. By injecting stem cells directly to the site of injury or inflammation inside the epidural space, doctors may drive tissue regeneration and control inflammatory responses, providing patients a route to long-term comfort and recovery.

Tissue Engineering: Building Bridges to Recovery

Tissue engineering technologies provide unique alternatives for repairing and rebuilding damaged tissues inside the epidural region, providing a scaffold for cell proliferation and tissue integration. By manufacturing biomimetic scaffolds consisting of biocompatible materials, researchers may generate conditions favorable to tissue regeneration, encouraging the infiltration of cells and the development of new tissue structures.

In the field of epidural anesthesia, tissue engineering shows promise for tackling a variety of clinical issues, from spinal cord injury to degenerative disc disease. By implanting biomaterial scaffolds filled with therapeutic drugs or stem cells into the epidural space, doctors may encourage tissue regeneration, reduce pain, and restore function, affording patients a road to recovery and enhanced quality of life.

16.3.3: Telemedicine and Remote Monitoring: Connecting Patients and Providers

Virtual Consultations: Expanding Access to Care

Telemedicine systems provide virtual access to specialist pain management treatments, linking patients with professional doctors regardless of geographic location. By employing video conferencing, telemedicine systems allow patients to consult with pain management professionals, get individualized treatment suggestions, and access educational materials from the comfort of their own homes.

In the arena of epidural anesthesia, video consultations provide a lifeline to patients in distant or underdeveloped locations, offering access to professional treatment and assistance that may otherwise be inaccessible. By providing virtual consultations, physicians can perform full evaluations, evaluate imaging tests, and build individualized treatment plans, ensuring that all patients get the care they need to manage their pain and maximize their results.

Wearable Devices: Empowering Patients in Their Journey to Recovery

Wearable devices paired with biosensors give a window into patients' physiological condition and pain levels, allowing continuous monitoring and remote control of postoperative pain. By wearing these devices, patients may measure their vital signs, activity levels, and pain ratings in real-time, offering significant insights into their recovery status and allowing early diagnosis of issues.

In the field of epidural anesthesia, wearable gadgets provide a method of empowering patients in their road to recovery, allowing them to actively engage in their treatment and monitor their progress from the comfort of their own homes. By wearing these devices, patients may connect with their healthcare providers, report changes in their symptoms, and get prompt treatments as required, ensuring that their pain is successfully controlled and their rehabilitation is maximized.

Conclusion: Embracing the Future of Epidural Anesthesia

The future of epidural anesthesia is overflowing with potential, as researchers and doctors alike start on a voyage of discovery and innovation. From precision medicine to regenerative medicines, telemedicine, and wearable technology, the possibilities are boundless. By embracing these future possibilities and utilizing the power of technology, we may usher in a new era of pain treatment, where every patient gets individualized care suited to their specific requirements and preferences.

As we navigate the route towards this future, it is vital to retain a consistent commitment to ethical practice, patient-centered care, and multidisciplinary teamwork. By working together, we can unleash the full potential of epidural anesthesia, improving the lives of patients and redefining the profession of pain management for centuries to come.

This part presents a detailed study of the future possibilities in epidural anesthesia, including insights into new trends, innovative ideas, and transformational technology set to revolutionize the landscape of pain management and perioperative care. Through a blend of creative thinking and imaginative foresight, we may chart the way towards a future where pain is controlled with accuracy, compassion, and humanity.